Fat Nation

Fat Nation

A History of Obesity in America

Jonathan Engel

ROWMAN & LITTLEFIELD
Lanham • Boulder • New York • London

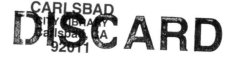

Published by Rowman & Littlefield
An imprint of The Rowman & Littlefield Publishing Group, Inc.
4501 Forbes Boulevard, Suite 200, Lanham, Maryland 20706
www.rowman.com

6 Tinworth Street, London SE11 5AL, United Kingdom

British Library Cataloguing in Publication Information Available

Library of Congress Cataloging-in-Publication Data
Names: Engel, Jonathan, author.
Title: Fat nation : a history of obesity in America / Jonathan Engel.
Description: Lanham, Maryland : Rowman & Littlefield, [2018] | Includes
  bibliographical references and index.
Identifiers: LCCN 2018043678 (print) | LCCN 2018043929 (ebook) |
  ISBN 9781538117750 (electronic) | ISBN 9781538117743 (cloth : alk. paper)
Subjects: | MESH: Obesity—history | History, 20th Century | History, 21st
  Century | United States
Classification: LCC RA645.O23 (ebook) | LCC RA645.O23 (print) | NLM WD 210 |
  DDC 362.1963/98—dc23
LC record available at https://lccn.loc.gov/2018043678

∞™ The paper used in this publication meets the minimum requirements of American National Standard for Information Sciences—Permanence of Paper for Printed Library Materials, ANSI/NISO Z39.48-1992.

Printed in the United States of America

MARCH 2019

Contents

1

An Old Problem

In 1952, the director of the National Institutes of Health (NIH), W. H. Sebrell Jr., announced that obesity was the "number one" nutritional problem in the United States, superseding malnutrition and vitamin deficiency.[1] Abundant harvests and falling food prices in recent years had erased the effects of the parsimony and rationing of the depression and war years, and Americans had dug into the bounty with gusto. Now they bore the cost of their gluttony, that "unlovely condition called corpulence," in the words of a 1926 testimony, which rendered its victims "comical" and "pitiable."[2] The condition was no laughing matter, noted David Barr, the chief of medicine at Cornell Medical School. Besides the usual scourges of diabetes, hypertension, arteriosclerosis, and heart failure, it was responsible for "maceration, intertrigo, eczema, and furunculosis . . . postural emphysema, flat feet, hernia, and osteoarthritis of the hips and knees." It was "unaesthetic, socially unacceptable, and psychologically crippling." It shortened life, undercut dignity, and eroded fortitude. For those who suffered its scourges, it shortened a life that had been made "ridiculous and miserable by its presence."[3]

The cause of the problem was disarmingly simple. In 1947, Hilde Bruch of Columbia University's Department of Psychiatry announced to the world that obesity was caused by overeating. (*Time* magazine deemed the insight "headline catching."[4]) Yet eating less was no small matter. Already, in the early 1950s, physicians were observing the futility of weight reduction. Eating less was a reasonable goal, yet most who attempted the feat were thwarted. Howard Rusk, the dean of American rehabilitative medicine, noted sadly in 1952 that most of the twenty-five million overweight Americans who resolved to lose a few pounds would "forget it as soon as they sit down to their next meal."[5] Indeed, in an age before labor-saving devices had aggressively sucked physical activity from the lives of most Americans and before multicar households obviated the need to walk and microwaves had replaced cooking with reheating, Americans were already finding that fat was a stubborn nemesis. "We're going to have to take off the kid gloves in dealing with people who are wallowing in their own grease," warned Edward Bortz, a Philadelphia physician.[6]

The problem had hardly started in 1952. As early as 1947 the United States Public Health Service (PHS) went hunting for undiagnosed diabetes in Oxford, Massachusetts (the birthplace of Clara Barton, founder of the Red Cross) and discovered, as suspected, that diabetes was sharply on the rise. Extrapolating from the Oxford findings, the PHS raised its estimate of diabetes cases in the nation from 1.5 million to 2.8 million.[7] In 1949, an NIH scientist, Edward Stieglitz, warned that obesity was a "national health problem ranking with tuberculosis in importance."[8] Through the 1950s and 1960s, a small number of public health officials and nutritionists watched, with alarm, as increasing numbers of Americans registered unhealthy weights. John Kelly Sr., the famed US Olympic single sculls oarsman, expressed alarm in 1955 that American youth was growing "softer, weaker, and flabbier." Lest action be taken, the United States would become, "a nation of weaklings."[9] In 1971, an editorial in the *New England Journal of Medicine* described the condition as "the most prevalent metabolic disorder of the age."[10] And by 1985, a sampling of grade school children subjected to the simple abdominal skin-pinch test found that both boys and girls were "significantly fatter" than children studied in the 1960s.[11] Another study, conducted the same year, found that more than a third of third- and fourth-grade children could not complete ten minutes of moderate exercise.[12]

The 1980s were a watershed decade for American obesity. Numbers had been rising gradually for decades, but from 1980 to 1995, the increase accelerated sharply. In that time, the portion of Americans who were "seriously overweight" jumped from a quarter of the population to a third. Fifty-eight million Americans weighed more than 20 percent above their ideal body weight, and the average American adult was eight pounds heavier than he or she had been at the beginning of the era.[13] Many

Americans recognized that they were growing fatter, and some even made efforts to reduce but to little effect. Over a third of adult women claimed to be on diets, yet virtually none could consistently keep weight off, even if they managed to temporarily shed pounds. John McCall, an endocrinologist in California, reflected, "The statistics are horrible. It's like treating cancer."[14] Indeed, seven years after losing weight, only 2 percent had managed to keep most of it off.

By 1998, 97 million adult Americans were overweight or obese, making it, by most measures, the fattest industrialized country in the world.[15] Two-thirds of all Americans were above their ideal weight.[16] The percentage of overweight adult men in the United States beat out British counterparts by a full 10 percent and even topped their Canadian neighbors.[17] Adults in every state and ethnic group were growing fatter, although the rise in the American Hispanic population was starker than most. The only good news was that men seemed to top out on the scales by about age of fifty, after which the portion of adult males who were overweight stabilized. Women had no such luck, however. They continued to get fatter for another fifteen years, and possibly longer.[18]

Perhaps more worrisome was the rapid rise in childhood obesity. During the same period of increase in adult obesity, childhood obesity rose 54 percent, and adolescent obesity rose 39 percent. The gains in obesity among African American children were even higher.[19] Furthermore, newer data belied the old myth that chubby children thinned out in adolescence and young adulthood. In fact, childhood obesity appeared to be highly correlated with adult obesity, and the earlier the problem started, the more intractable it seemed to be.

Childhood obesity was wrought from the same two causes as adult obesity—inactivity and overeating—but seemed to be particularly compounded by television watching. Data collected in the 1990s repeatedly pointed to television as a particularly noxious culprit in producing chubby kids, even while holding household income and education constant.[20] One of the few groups of kids in the country who were not getting fat, despite eating a fairly high-calorie diet, were Amish children, who eschewed television along with cell phones and cars. Amish kids burned calories just walking between farms to see their friends and had to rely on face-to-face contact to communicate. Alan Shuldiner, a researcher at the University of Maryland, noted, "You never see obese Amish children. Never."[21] Children also appeared to be particularly susceptible to food marketing and portion size. Many pediatricians noted that they could not recall seeing children overeating in the past; most seemed to have an innate braking mechanism on their appetites. One pediatrician who worked on portion size noted the novel "disinhibition" he was seeing for the first time in children's eating habits. "I never saw children who ate and ate and ate until you finally had to cut them off," he related.[22]

Rising obesity in children was bringing the same toxic mix of type II diabetes, high blood pressure, metabolic syndrome, and fatty liver that it did in adults, although cardiac and vascular symptoms tended to hold off until later years. It also brought social isolation, anxiety, and depression. Fat children were more likely to drop out of high school, less likely to finish college, less likely to marry, and less likely to earn high incomes. The risk of dying by middle age was two to three times higher for obese adolescent girls than for their healthy-weight peers. One research team estimated that childhood obesity would shorten life expectancy in the United States by five years within a generation.[23] Another team estimated that each additional pound of weight above the ideal brought a 2 percent increase in death.[24]

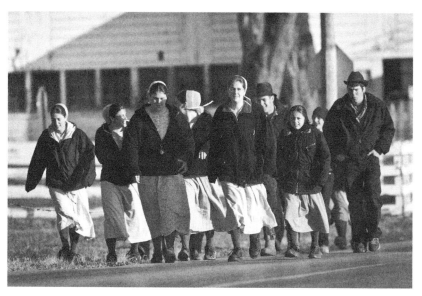

Amish children are almost never fat, despite eating diets relatively high in sugar, fat, and carbohydrates. The secret is constant movement: particularly walking. The Amish culture prohibits the use of motorized vehicles. *Planetpix/Alamy Stock Photo*

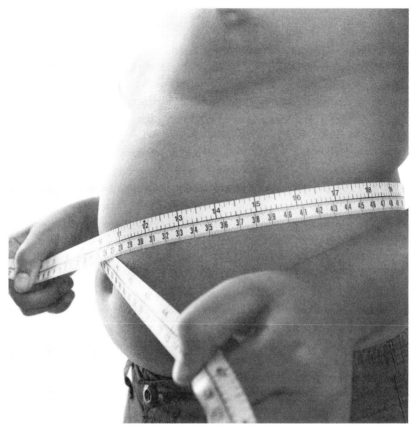

The most sobering aspect of the American obesity epidemic has been the rapid increase in the number of overweight and obese children and teenagers. *Getty Images*

Of greatest concern was the rise in type II diabetes. This insidious disease, previously so unknown in children as to earn the sobriquet "adult-onset diabetes," had increased tenfold in adolescents during this period. Unlike type I diabetes in which the pancreas simply produces no insulin, type II diabetes results from the body's tissues growing insensitive to the catalytic action of insulin. The body produces large amounts of the hormone, but the hormone cannot move glucose—the body's essential fuel—into muscle cells for metabolism, or into fat cells for storage. Rather, the glucose stays in the blood where it works perniciously over decades to destroy organs and clog capillaries. Long-time sufferers frequently go blind, lose kidney and liver function, and lose limbs to gangrene and amputation.[25]

The costs of the phenomenon were immense. As far back as 1946, physicians recognized the high rates of hypertension, cardiac disease, joint disease, and diabetes associated with fat. Armed with tremendous amounts of demographic and health data from the wartime draft, physicians were able to pinpoint excessive intake of refined starches as a cause of liver disease.[26] In 1952, Louis Dublin, the chief statistician of the Metropolitan Life Insurance Company, along with his colleagues published results of actuarial calculations performed on thousands of army officers and industrial workers showing that hypertension was two and a half times more common among obese individuals as it was among individuals of normal weight. The same researchers showed that arterial disease was more than three times as common in the heavier group and that type II diabetes was nearly twenty times as common.[27] Both overweight men and women physically fell more frequently, reported more absences from work, and recovered more slowly from surgery. Overweight women reported more problems during pregnancy and childbirth and had higher rates of gestational diabetes. Heavy people had more kidney and gallbladder disease. Babies born to heavy mothers tended to be heavy themselves, and the children were more prone to diabetes later in life. One pithy internist noted that "two-thirds of his income would be cut off if people ate properly."[28]

In later decades, scientists refined their conclusions about the ills of obesity and quantified the dangers, but they hardly retracted their conclusions. If anything, obesity seemed to be more dangerous than scientists in the 1950s had supposed. For example, by 1985, oncologists and nutritionists had found that obese women were more likely to die from cancer of the gallbladder, ovaries, breast, and uterus, while obese men were more likely than their slim counterparts to die from cancer of the colon and prostate. In that year, William Castelli, director of the famed Framingham Heart Study, was able to state that over a period of twenty-six years, mortality rates in a studied population rose by 2 percent for each pound an individual was over his or her ideal weight. One observer could only conclude from the research that "obesity kills."[29]

By 2004, the costs in lost earnings, medical bills, and suffering due to obesity were stratospheric. Obesity was costing the nation $150 billion annually in medical expenditures, and the cost in lost wages was incalculable.[30] Amazingly, obesity was poised to surpass smoking as the nation's worst preventable killer, with the number of deaths associated with "poor diet and physical inactivity" just brushing the 435,000 deaths caused each year by tobacco.[31] Obesity killed, and its rate of killing could only increase.

As bad as the physical costs of obesity were, however, the psychological and social costs were almost worse. Obese people faced being socially ostracized, ridiculed, and discriminated against. Obese children found themselves marginalized at school and excluded from sports. One overweight teenager remembered how she would sometimes be invited to parties "just for laughs" and described a mortifying incident in which she was plunked into a trash basket and, unable to get out, was rolled down a hill.[32] Obesity in girls often fell along class lines, thus further differentiating the rich from the poor. A 1986 study found that while 30 percent of lower-class women were obese, only 5 percent upper-class ones were.[33] One psychologist writing in 1957 noted that "the overweight teenager is doomed to the role of wallflower at parties and to go through school dateless." And social discrimination from same-sex peers was hardly less cruel.[34] One study had children view pictures of kids with various physical deformities, including being fat, and asked the participants which child they would like to have as their friend. The fat children were rated lowest.[35] Not surprisingly, overweight children and teenagers tended to be disproportionately depressed and to show evidence of truncated or distorted social development. Frederick Werkman, a psychiatric researcher, wrote of the way in which these kids' lives were "seriously distorted."[36]

Obese people faced discrimination at all ages and junctures. A series of studies showed that overweight men applying to selective colleges were half as likely to be accepted as their non-overweight counterparts, while overweight women were *one-third* as likely to be admitted.[37] Employers were, if anything, even more biased against hiring overweight women, telling obese applicants that they were unacceptable regardless of their qualifications. In 1985, Catherine McDermott successfully sued Xerox for withdrawing a job offer after learning of her height and weight because she would be "an assault to the eyes of the director" (in her words).[38] And both overweight men and women, even when hired, related being regularly passed over for promotions.

There was no great mystery as to why Americans had been steadily gaining weight since the end of World War II: They ate too much and moved too little. As early as the immediate post-war years, public health leaders warned of the dangers of overly large portion sizes—particularly carbohydrates. Thomas Desmond, who chaired multiple health-oriented committees while serving in the New York State Senate, wrote the following in 1949: "We push more than four pounds of bread or equivalent cakes into our stomachs each week. We fill up on 2.3 pounds of potatoes weekly. We're eating more meat than we did before World War II and are loading ourselves with about 3,400 calories a day compared with 3,250 caloric burden before the war. . . . Sure, stuff yourself with bread, load up with potatoes, dump spoonfuls of sugar into your coffee, fill up with rich puddings—but be prepared for the consequences."[39]

Moreover, Americans were moving less and less each year. While it was true that exercise could only make a scant impact on obesity (an hour of semi-vigorous exercise only burned about 300 calories or a little over an ounce of fat), more movement was better than less. But suburbanization, the rise of the auto culture, shopping malls, unwalkable towns, gadgets, labor-saving devices, and even remote controls all diminished the already modest amount of activity most Americans performed daily. While the running craze of the 1970s and the aerobics trend of the 1980s had induced some of the upper middle class to exercise more frequently, the numbers were hardly promising. The most common activity in America in 1985 was swimming, in which 41 percent of Americans participated at least *once per year*. Fishing, at 34 percent, was a distant second, and so it went from there. George Harris, the editor of *American Health*, summed it up nicely: "The evidence shows that we are a bunch of fat slobs who do not have activity built into our daily lives."[40] By that year, a typical American teenager spent thirteen hours per week in physical motion but over forty hours per week watching television and playing video games. The Amateur Athletic Union reported that the percentage of children passing its basic standard for pushups, high jump, long jump, and running had dropped from 42 percent to 30 percent in just a few years.

What had happened? How had a minor public health nuisance, always present but never threatening, ballooned into the single greatest health threat in the industrialized world in just two generations? Had people lost their resolve? Had the essential American character corroded? Or had some odd but toxic confluence of lifestyle changes, eating habits, available foodstuffs, and social mores all conspired to undermine the basic homeostatic mechanisms by which people's bodies regulated food intake and weight?

In 2014, the US government reported a fragment of good news about the epidemic: obesity rates in very young children (under the age of five) appeared to be leveling off, albeit at a very high level. Most Americans, though, continued to get fatter, and death rates for middle-aged white men were climbing alarmingly.[41] At the same time, new research performed by psychologists and behavioral economists demonstrated that most people had less control over their impulses and urges than they thought, particularly around food. The answer seemed to derive from a changing environment, changing life patterns, changing foodstuffs, changing eating habits, a changing family structure, and changing work norms. By 2015, the life of a typical middle-class American was so profoundly distant from the life of his nineteenth-century forebears that virtually every aspect of his day seemed reasonable ground to explore in understanding obesity. This book attempts to do just that.

2

Whence Cometh Fat?

A THRIFTY ANIMAL

We evolved to be fat. With our enormous brains, hunter-gatherer feeding strategies, and social impulses, human bodies diverged from those of other primates some 100,000 years ago to become rounder, softer, and lazier. A newborn human baby uses 60 percent of its daily calories just to keep its brain functioning, and with its small stomach and twitchy gut, it needs to feed five to six times daily to adequately ingest those calories. To supply those hungry infants, and to gestate them during pregnancy, adult women are between 20 and 25 percent pure fat in even the slimmest societies. Adult males are slimmer, at roughly 10 percent fat, but even they substantially out-lard most of our closest primate relatives. Chimps and baboons, for example, are born with 3 percent body fat and top out at about 6 percent as adults.[1] And lest you think that this tendency is new, the famously chunky *Venus of Willendorf*, a statue of a morbidly obese woman, is at least 20,000 years old.[2]

We evolved to store fat rapidly because as hunter-gatherers our lot was feast or famine. Walking ten to fourteen miles each day, adult males traversed the savannah in search of the rare kill that could feed an entire family group. When food was available, people overindulged and put on excess weight that would sustain them through scarcity. They evolved special digestive processes to metabolize the starchy roots and fruits that made up the balance of their diets and convert it efficiently to fat—so

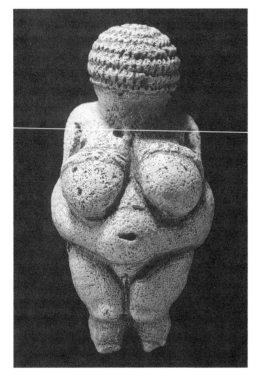

The *Venus of Willendorf*, dating back 20,000 years. A few people have always been obese, but only recently has the problem become pervasive. *Getty Images*

efficiently that humans have been called starch specialists.[3] With our long legs and pendular strides, we became hyper-efficient locomotors: among the most energy efficient in the animal kingdom. Humans are lousy runners relative to other large mammals—the fastest among us tops out at about thirty miles per hour, which is slower than a middling giraffe—but we are amazingly efficient walkers. More than one dieter has realized with dismay that her five-mile hike burned no more calories than could be replaced by one good-sized chocolate chip cookie. Fortunately for our waistlines, food was often scarce, distances in the savannah were vast, and most prey eluded us easily.

Fast-forward 50,000 years and we find ourselves the victims of our own evolution. Today's sedentary office worker burns only about 750 calories during the course of her workday: about half of what a factory worker burned fifty years ago, and about a sixth of what a coal miner, sod cutter, or lumberjack burned fifty years before that.[4] Our extraordinary legs, designed to effortless carry us ten, fifteen, even twenty miles daily, now go unused; the typical American adult walks less than *one-third* of one mile per day. Elevators have replaced stairs, ubiquitous electronic and gas transport have replaced ambulation, and power tools have eased every task from ditch-digging to beating eggs. Indeed, in the past generation, we have ceased to roll down our own car windows, rise from the couch to change television channels, or even walk behind a power mower. The three authors of *The Paleolithic Prescription* argue, pithily, that we lived as hunter-gatherers for 100,000 generations, as agriculturists for 500 generations, as industrialists for ten, and as post-industrialists for one.[5] Our thrifty genes cannot evolve anywhere near fast enough to accommodate these extraordinary changes in our lifestyle.[6]

Moreover, unlikely as it might seem, we evolved to be *lazy*.[7] Like all hunting mammals, our bodies are designed for limited periods of exertion, followed by long periods of rest. We power down during the cold, dark months of winter, not quite hibernating but sleeping more, moving less, and generally conserving our energy. We succumb to the heat of the day during summer months, taking refuge in the shade for multihour naps. Indeed, most of us find it counterintuitive to move our bodies when we do not have to. Designers of shopping malls know to limit sight lines in corridors to no more than seventy-five yards, lest shoppers get discouraged at

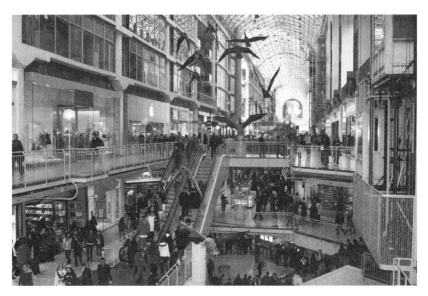

Modern shopping malls are carefully constructed with limited sight lines. Developers know that few Americas will walk more than seventy-five yards. *Getty Images*

the walking challenge and head home. Although nutritionists endlessly remind us of the health benefits derived from even modest amounts of daily exercise, few of us can override our natural indolence to accomplish this. In 2012, the Centers for Disease Control and Prevention (CDC) estimated that 80 percent of Americans did not manage to exercise at moderate intensity for 2.5 hours per *week*—about twenty minutes per day.[8]

FAT IS COMPLICATED

If being less heavy were simply a matter of eating less and moving more, we might have made more progress against obesity. But the more we study fat, the more complicated it appears to be. There is more to fat than meets the eye, and not all fat is the same.

Fat is stored in fat cells (adipocytes), which are primarily laid down in infancy. In the first few years of life, the number of fat cells increases in response to caloric intake. That is, overfed babies actually produce more fat cells that are capable of storing fat later in life. Once the fat cells are created, they can grow and shrink in response to caloric input and output, but they never go away. One study of dieting women found that they could reduce their fat cells to normal size relatively easily, but shrinking them further brought upon nearly uncontrollable urges to eat.[9]

In fact, the news is even worse. Recent research has shown that a fetus can respond to the uterine environment by developing more adipocytes than we would normally expect to see. Undernourished pregnant women tend to produce babies with more fat cells that are then more prone to obesity later in life. It is as if the baby's body, responding to a nutrient-scarce environment, prepares itself for a lifetime of scarcity by becoming hypervigilant at storing fat.[10] Once the baby is outside the womb, however, the body reverses and starts creating more fat cells in response to food surplus rather than food scarcity. In studies done of overfed human babies in the late 1960s, researchers found that fat cell counts in obese children were substantially higher than in normal-weight children.[11]

Our primate cousins develop similarly. In the early 1980s, a group of researchers in San Antonio, Texas, fed baby baboons 40 percent more calories in infant formula than they would have received through normal breastfeeding. By the time these overfed baboons were five years old (roughly equivalent to a human teenager), their bodies were 28 percent fat, as compared to baboons in control groups who were only 7 percent fat.[12]

Fat cells are remarkably elastic, capable of swelling to many times their normal size when engorged with triglycerides—the fatty acid chains which make up human fat tissue. At the same time, they appear to be more than simply passive fat vessels. Adipose tissue can signal brain and gastro-intestinal receptors to eat more or less to maintain a certain preset size. Researchers who remove fat cells from obese mice find that the remaining fat cells have a tendency to maintain their previous size, despite the fact that the mice are now substantially thinner. More troubling, however, is the fact that people who have been obese since childhood maintain their many fat cells—as many as three times normal—even after losing substantial amounts of weight. In one study, researchers at Rockefeller University found that previously obese women who had lost substantial amounts of weight appeared to be physiologically starving, despite being at a healthy weight. They ceased to menstruate, lost white blood cells, and complained of cold and hunger. They became obsessed with food. One science writer reporting on the women noted that they looked like people with anorexia nervosa.[13] We can shrink our fat cells, but we cannot kill them off.

Human fat comes in two colors: yellow and brown. We store our yellow, or subcutaneous, fat in our rears and thighs, and we store our brown, or visceral, fat (also called brown adipose tissue or BAT) in our abdomens. Of the two, abdominal fat is substantially more dangerous, as it is more metabolically active. Abdominal fat, also known as a paunch or a "beer belly," is highly correlated with greater risk of heart disease, high blood pressure, and general inflammation. Subcutaneous fat, by contrast, is largely inert. Women with big rumps but relatively flat stomachs are about as healthy as their skinnier colleagues. However, just a few extra pounds of abdominal fat can be deadly.

Brown fat cells are much larger than yellow fat cells, and they rapidly throw off fatty acids that interfere with insulin processing. Brown fat cells are proximate to the liver (by way of the portal vein) where those fatty acids can interfere with the liver's metabolism of insulin and cause a spike in insulin levels and can induce the liver to produce triglycerides, raising levels of bad (LDL) cholesterol. Brown fat is toxic enough that even when it is not visually evident, its presence in the abdominal cavity can wreak havoc on the liver and pancreas. Japanese men, in particular, manifest the odd syndrome of being thin on the outside and fat on the inside ("TOFI," for thin-outside-fat-inside, in endocrinological speak) wherein despite being of normal weight and girth, they exhibit symptoms of fatty liver disease and metabolic disorder. (This will be discussed further in Chapter

6.) On the plus side, brown fat responds rapidly to dieting and is the first fat that is lost when people begin losing weight. Decreasing brown fat reserves by only a few pounds can make a profound difference in the heart health of obese people.[14] Yellow fat, to the consternation of many middle-aged women, is far more resistant to dieting and tends to stick around even in austere environments.

Brown fat is dangerous in other ways too. It appears to depress the production of high-density lipoproteins (HDLs), the "good cholesterol" that the body uses to clear plaque from the bloodstream and maintain good arterial health. At times, simply measuring a patient's waist-to-hip ratio (WHR) is a reasonable predictor of HDL levels in the blood.[15] Brown fat tends to grow with elevated cortisol that accompanies stress. Stress really *is* dangerous to your health.[16]

This yellow/brown fat dichotomy has been known to researchers since as far back as 1949 when actuaries at Metropolitan Life found that men with waist measurements only two inches larger than normal were at a 50 percent increased risk of heart attack.[17] Research in the 1950s found that "apple-shaped" women (with substantial amounts of abdominal fat) were far more likely to suffer from atherosclerosis and diabetes than "pear-shaped" women, despite weighing the same,[18] and researchers in Sweden found that people with large stomachs were three to five times as likely to have heart attacks as thin-waisted compatriots.[19] The Swedish researchers, looking at thousands of different subjects, were even able to put a precise measurement on the danger ratio. For men, a waist-to-hip ratio over 1.0 was enough to put them in the danger zone; for women, the ratio could not go over 0.8.

Brown fat burns hot. In mammals, the adipose tissue is metabolized in a highly exothermic reaction that allows individuals to raise their body temperature in response to cold. This is one of the ways in which bears and other hibernating mammals maintain body temperature in the cold of winter while remaining nearly perfectly still. Although at less than 1 percent of body weight in most healthy people, brown fat at times is responsible for half of all of the heat generated by the body.[20] For people prone to obesity, the brown fat seems to lack this capacity, or at least burns ineffectively. It is not uncommon to hear obese people complain about feeling cold, even though intuition might suggest that their subcutaneous fat could insulate their bodies against the cold. Their insulation may be intact, but they have a faulty pilot light and cannot ignite their brown fat burners to stay warm.[21]

Everything about fat, both abdominal and subcutaneous, is sticky. Multiple studies have shown that fat children become fat adults and that the adults are fat in the same way as they were fat as children. One of the earliest public health studies, performed on school children in Hagerstown, Maryland, in the late 1930s, found that of fifty overweight boys, 86 percent were overweight as adults and that of fifty overweight girls, 80 percent were overweight as adults. For the normal-weight boys and girls, only 42 percent and 18 percent, respectively, were heavy as adults.[22] Perhaps more disturbing is that overweight pregnant women tend to give birth to babies who are, themselves, likely to be fat as adults, and who will go on to develop diabetes at rates seven times the normal rate.[23] Multiple studies over the years have established this high correlation between juvenile and adult obesity, and the pattern seems to be as firmly set today as it was when the first studies were done in the 1930s.[24] The US Army, which tends to like its soldiers trim and healthy, has long known of the relationship between youthful obesity and middle-aged diabetes and heart disease. Moreover, even when people do lose weight during middle-age, they tend to stay the same shape; apples stay apples, and pears stay pears. Rudolph Leibel of Rockefeller University noted, "While we may be able to shrink in size, changing our proportions through dieting may be nearly impossible."[25]

The bacteria in our gut further complicates the scenario. The billions of bacteria that live symbiotically in our intestines are critical to proper digestion. In particular, these bacteria, collectively known as the human *biome*, break up fermenting soluble fiber into short-chain fatty acids, which produce roughly 10 percent of our energy. Different people have biomes that are more or less effective at this task. You might think that people with biomes that digest fiber poorly would be thinner, given that the human gut cannot absorb energy from fiber that has not been fermented by the bacteria. However, the opposite appears to be true. The short-chain fatty acids produced by a healthy biome do produce more calories for the body, but they also act as an important mechanism to signal satiation. Incidentally, bacterial activity in the gut produces a lot of flatulence as a by-product, which turns out to be the mark of both a healthy, fiber-rich diet and a healthy biome. David Lustig, a prominent obesity researcher, pithily notes that our choice comes down to "fart or fat."

We kill off these bacteria at our own peril. Overuse of antibiotics in infants and children can distort the natural biome and induce obesity.[26] Ranchers have long known that adding antibiotics to cattle-feed produces substantially fatter cows. Feeding antibiotics to mice in a laboratory does the same thing, generating mice that are 25 percent fatter.[27] We do not know precisely which bacteria are the good ones and which are the bad ones, but the correlation is clear. One study of Danes found that obese individuals had only a little more than half of the bacterial gene variety in their stool as normal weight individuals.[28]

Interestingly, we can actually take good bacteria and transplant them into the guts of people with poor biomes through fecal transplants. (Yes, it's exactly what it sounds like.) Fat mice that have had their biomes killed off with antibiotics become thin again when they have healthy bacteria transferred to their guts, and fat people do too.[29] People feel less hungry when they have good bacteria in their guts, provided that they eat a high-fiber diet. They fart more too, but we may all just have to get over that.[30]

GENETIC SIGNALING

Although we are regularly told that our eating habits are under our conscious control, a good deal of research over the past half-century indicates otherwise. As far back as 1910, at least a few physicians admitted that obesity seemed to run in families.[31] Ethnologists and anthropologists have long observed that some isolated ethnic groups have specific body types that predominate, despite eating similar diets as nearby tribes whose bodies might appear quite different. Pima Indians, for example, in the American Southwest, are obese at levels far more than other localized populations, as are Mennonites, Old Order Amish, and natives of the Island of Kosrae. Moreover, while Americans are generally fatter than citizens of other countries, certain ethnic populations in the United States seem to respond to our obesogenic environment by gaining weight even more rapidly than most Americans, among them immigrants from Mexico and West Africa.

Some of the earliest insights into the genetic roots of obesity grew out of work conducted in the late 1940s at Jackson Memorial Laboratory in Bar Harbor, Maine. There, researchers found that certain strains of mice grew fatter than normal—more than doubling the weight of their cousins at thirty weeks. These mice preferred food that was high in fat content, in contrast to most mice that preferred protein-dense but low-fat food. When the mice were injected with thyroid hormone, they lost weight rapidly. Researchers also found that if they removed the pituitary gland from obese mice, the mice also lost weight rapidly. It appeared that some feedback mechanism that allowed the pituitary gland to maintain a normal weight in the mice did not function correctly.[32]

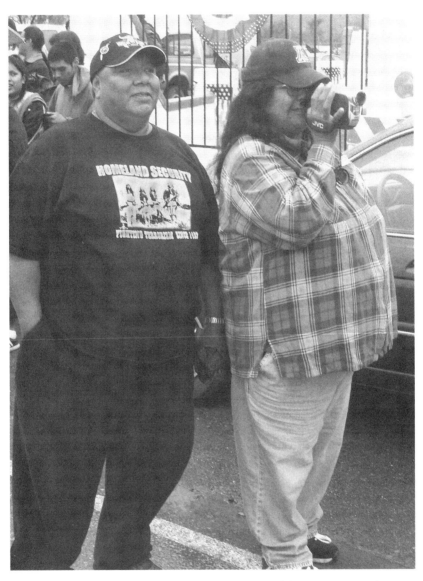

Obesity has a strong genetic component. Pima Indians of the American Southwest have rapidly become obese in the presence of a Western diet. *Pixels.Com/ David Lee Guss*

Ten years later, Douglas Coleman, working at the same lab, started a series of macabre experiments with two different types of abnormal mice: ones that were abnormally fat, which he labeled as *ob* mice, and ones that had a congenital propensity to diabetes, which he labeled *db* mice (they were also unusually fat). Reasoning that the *ob* and *db* mice were missing some sort of hormone or protein, he tried surgically binding them to normal littermates, creating a series of conjoined mice. What he found surprised him: When he joined a *db* mouse with a normal mouse, the normal mouse stopped eating and, ultimately, starved to death. However, when he joined an *ob* mouse with a normal mouse, the *ob* mouse lost weight and became of normal weight. Coleman reasoned that the *db* mice were making large amounts of an appetite-suppressing hormone but that their brains were insensitive to it. When normal mice were bound to them, however, the normal mice's brains were sensitive to the hormone, and they stopped eating. The *ob* mice, by contrast, were not making the hormone but were sensitive to it. When they were bound to normal mice, the hormone entered their bloodstream and worked on receptors in their brains to suppress their appetites. The question was then why were certain mice missing the ability to either make the appetite-suppressing hormone or be sensitive to it.

Other researchers found additional evidence that people's eating habits were being controlled as much by their hormones as by their conscious decisions. In 1967, Ethan Sims experimented with prisoners at the Vermont State Prison to see how their bodies responded to intentional gluttony. A group of twenty prisoners agreed to eat 10,000 calories per day over a period of days: roughly four times their typical caloric need. The prisoners, as expected, gained weight, but most had trouble maintaining the new higher weight, and upon reverting to a normal diet, they each almost lost all of the weight they had gained. Two prisoners, however, gained weight rapidly on the new diet and even upon the cessation of the diet had a very difficult time returning to their old weight. It was as if their bodies *wanted* to get fat. Both of these men admitted to coming from families with a history of obesity.[33]

Even more telling was the work conducted by Albert Stunkard in the 1980s on adopted children in Denmark. Studying 540 adoptees, Stunkard's team found that their adult weights more closely paralleled the weights of their biological parents than their adoptive parents, suggesting that their genes were more dispositive in determining their adult weights than the culture and households in which they had been raised. In fact, 80 percent of the adoptees who had two obese biological parents became obese themselves, as opposed to 14 percent of adoptees who had two normal-weight parents.[34] Stunkard found additional evidence for genetic roots of obesity by studying 4,000 sets of male twins who had served in the US Army during World War II and the Korean War. Roughly half of the twin sets were fraternal, and half were identical. The research team found substantially higher concordance in bodyweight and obesity between the identical twins than between the fraternal twins. It appeared that 80 percent of the variation in bodyweight was produced by genetic effects.[35] In a separate study, a team led by Claude Bouchard at Laval University in Quebec deliberately overfed twelve pairs of identical twins 1,000 calories a day for three months. By the end of the period, the participants had gained varying amounts of weight, but notably, each set of twins tended to gain about the same amount of weight. That is, despite all being overfed the same amount of calories, the participants' bodies seemed to be genetically programmed to either store the additional energy or to burn it off through a higher metabolism.[36]

In 1994, scientists at the Howard Hughes Medical Institute and at Rockefeller University, led by Jeffrey Friedman, succeeded in identifying the gene responsible for the *ob* mice, which they named the *ob* gene. The gene, which codes for a specific protein, now known as leptin, malfunctions in the *ob* mice, and therefore their bodies cannot signal to their brains (to the hypothalamus specifically) that they are full. When these scientists, working in conjunction with scientists at Hoffman-La Roche and Amgen, injected the obese mice with artificially produced leptin, the mice ate less, burned more calories, and rapidly lost weight.

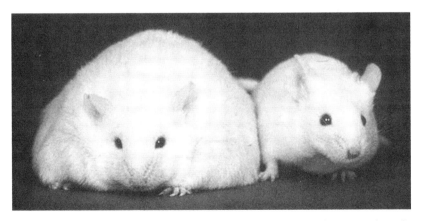

A good deal of our modern understanding of the action of leptin has come through rats that are genetically insensitive to it, or fail to produce it. The rat on the left above carries the *ob* gene. *Pixels.Com/David Lee Guss*

Our understanding of the genetic roots of obesity continues to evolve. Today we know of five different strains of genetically obese mice—known as yellow, fat, obese, diabetes, and tubby—the last being of particular interest to obesity researchers, as they tend to gain weight in the same way that people do: gradually and increasingly with age. Interestingly, tubby mice also have a difficult time making use of their insulin and tend to develop hearing and sight problems while young.[37]

Moreover, our understanding of the complexity of the body's feedback mechanisms to govern hunger, satiation, fat storage, and metabolism continues to grow. We now know of at least six feedback molecules and systems that work to maintain the body's weight. Leptin, for example, works closely with insulin—the body's central catalyst for moving glucose in and out of cells, and for storing the glucose as fat or burning it as energy. Both leptin and insulin find receptive sites on the hypothalamus, a gland at the base of the brain, which then signals satiety. At the same time, other hormones and molecules—Cholecystokinin (CCK) and Neuropeptide Y (NPY)—respond to weight loss by stimulating appetite. CCK, in turn, has an agonist molecule, CCK8, which negates the stimulating properties of CCK, while NPY works in conjunction with corticotrophin-releasing hormone (CRH) to stimulate food uptake. Notably, NPY secretion is stimulated by stress hormones such as corticosteroids. When we feel stress, we are driven to eat and to rapidly put on weight. This is one of the many reasons why it is easier to lose weight when you are relaxed, at ease, and working less hard.

The systems continue to get more complex. Recently, we have begun to explore the role of opiomelanocortin peptides, themselves precursors to endorphin formation—the body's natural opiates. Endorphins play a role in obesity, suggesting that we often eat to produce feelings of euphoria, and we cease to eat when we can achieve happiness in other ways. There is a reason that heroin addicts have little trouble keeping their weight down.

SET POINTS

To a large degree, our bodies appear to have a preferred weight and are able to defend that weight. Unconsciously, or subconsciously, we modulate our base metabolic rates; eat more or less; move more or less; and experience greater degrees of hunger or satiety, all in an effort to maintain a preordained weight. Rats that have half of their fat cells surgically removed wind up at the same weight; the remaining fat cells simply swell to twice their previous size.[38] Nutritionists point out that if we overeat by only 200 calories per day—about one medium-size cookie—while maintaining steady metabolic and activity levels, we would gain twenty pounds in a year. Few of us can so accurately monitor our food intake, and yet most of us end the year only a few pounds above or below where we started. To put this in a different light, we typically eat about ten million calories in a decade. If we gained only ten pounds in that decade—a not uncommon weight gain in midlife—it would imply accuracy in calorie counting to about one-tenth of 1 percent daily.[39] Clearly, our bodies are slowing down and speeding up various processes to allow us to maintain a relatively constant weight over time.

As I've already pointed out, the body has a variety of complex feedback mechanisms designed to increase and decrease a feeling of hunger. Fat cells, the pancreas, the gut, the brain, and the liver all communicate with each other through various messenger molecules to open and shut off the hunger urge. One science writer vividly described fat cells as "sniffing the blood for traces of dessert, ever ready to send a squall of protest brainward if they sense deprivation."[40] Another medical writer pointed out that during times of deprivation, fat cells appear to hijack portions of the unconscious brain, "which can as easily desire fat as the conscious brain can yearn to possess an original Picasso."[41]

One reason we suspect that the body defends a set weight is by watching what happens to obese people as they lose weight by dieting. Invariably, their base metabolism drops as they approach their target weight, and they are forced to eat progressively fewer calories each day to maintain their new, svelter figures. One study of dieters by Overeaters Anonymous found that while many of them appeared to be of normal weight, many of their internal signs appeared as if they were starving. Their fat cells were tiny, their pulse and blood pressure were depressed, and many women had ceased to menstruate. They were frequently cold. "They were always thinking about food," noted Jules Hirsch, a researcher at Rockefeller University.[42] Moreover, Hirsch found that people who had lost and gained weight repeatedly, so-called "yo-yo" dieters, found it increasingly difficult to lose weight. Even when they returned to their previous weight, their bodies no longer needed as many calories to maintain that weight as they once did. It was as if the bodies had gone into a permanent starvation mode.

These patterns are observed even in babies, with overweight babies generating less body heat than normal-weight babies. One study comparing babies of overweight and normal-weight mothers found that children of overweight mothers burned 21 percent fewer calories at rest at the age of three months than did children of normal-weight mothers. These children just seemed to be born with a lower "idle."[43] Studies conducted by Clifton Bogardus of the Pima Indians found that nearly 70 percent of individuals in the tribe had unusually low metabolic rates, as measured by at-rest oxygen consumption.[44] In one terribly pessimistic study, Stunkard and colleagues estimated the chance of an obese adolescent becoming a normal-weight adult at 1 to 28.[45]

Heavy people don't just have a lower idle; they also unconsciously eat and move differently than normal-weight people, even from an early age. Overweight infants spend longer suckling, consume more milk from bottles before pushing the bottle away, and eat more solid food. Overweight mice, when given a choice, choose foods higher in fat content than their normal-weight littermates. As early as 1952, nutritionist Jean Mayer began to try to dispel the myth that overweight was merely a matter of willpower and poor eating habits. "There is certainly no evidence whatsoever that there is *not* a hereditary characteristic," he argued.[46]

Perhaps even more sobering have been the studies of motion, showing that thinner people simply *move* more than heavy people throughout their lives. Thinner people fidget more, wiggle their feet and legs more, and find reasons throughout the day to get up from their chairs to move.[47] Studies of obese girls in high school gym classes find that when participating in gym class, they conserve their motions to burn fewer calories than their thinner classmates, even while playing the same sports. Slim girls playing tennis and softball moved two and a half times as far during a class as heavier girls.[48] Studies of housewives in the 1960s found that leaner women walked twice as far each day as heavier ones, even when engaged in similar homemaking activities. Using stop-action photography in two co-ed summer camps in the 1970s, Jean Mayer and colleagues found that many of the heavier children expended virtually *no* calories while playing volleyball, tennis, and water sports. The girls dutifully showed up for the activity and then essentially stood still or free-floated in the water.[49] Not surprisingly, multiple studies of obese and normal-weight mice, fed the same diet, show that normal-weight mice run three times farther on an exercise wheel than their heavier cage-mates each day.[50]

This idea of inherent preferences in both eating and moving is consistent with our observations of people who lose weight in regimented situations. Everybody is capable of moving more and burning greater amounts of fat, but some people inherently prefer to move more while others prefer to move less. When placed in a regimented situation, such as in military training or under the tutelage of an all-absorbing obesity clinic, everybody can lose weight. The challenge arises when the regimentation is removed.[51] This also helps to explain why weight-loss programs with a social component, such as Weight Watchers, are more successful than solo programs, and why people with thinner friends are more likely to maintain lower weights than people with heavier friends. In the absence of a strong internal impulse toward slimming behavior, outside cues and pressures become far more important.

We are all fatter today (or most of us, anyway), so how does this fit with set-point theory? If set points are largely genetically determined, we would not expect to see a substantial change in average weights over relatively short periods of time. The answer, as I will repeatedly argue in the next few chapters, is that our environment has changed radically over the past century (particular the last half-century) such that many of the structural restraints around us that historically kept us from indulging our natural urge to eat more and move less are no longer present. Historically, food shortages or high food prices prevented many of us from eating as much as we may have wanted. At the same time, the necessity of physical effort to hunt, farm, or ranch prevented many of us from indulging our preference for indolence. Most of these restraints no longer exist. Calories are now ubiquitous and nearly free, while mechanized transport and physically non-taxing jobs allow many of us to go through our days in metabolic states that differ little from lying on a couch. We have been allowed to indulge our worst impulses to our own detriment.

3

The Unwalkable Landscape

AN UNWALKABLE LANDSCAPE

We have drastically rebuilt our environment since our days as hunter-gatherers, but for most of our history, we relied on our legs for transportation. Through different eras, people lived within walkable distances to a farm, trading post, factory, or office. Farms gathered closely around villages; cities clustered around ports. Overland travel was a regrettable hazard of the postal service and peddlers and few others. Most goods and materials were produced locally. Bringing building supplies from afar was so rare and extraordinary that the Bible explicitly mentions the "cedars of Lebanon" that Solomon had shipped in for his temple.

Walkability was not merely necessary; from a health standpoint, it was desirable. Our bodies are built to walk, and walking is the single best source of exercise and revitalization for the majority of the world's population. Walking is pleasant and social; requires neither training nor equipment; and is sustainable. Most people through history have been capable walkers until nearly the day that they died.

Walking is also the most likely path to weight control in our obesogenic world. Japanese children, among the world's thinnest, not incidentally walk to school at the highest rates. Nearly 99 percent of Japanese children walk to and from school, and the schools are placed so as to be walkable, in compliance with a "Walking to School Practice" policy in place since 1953.[1] Notably, the few areas Japan has seen a rise in childhood obesity have tended to be rural areas where schools cannot be feasibly placed within walkable distances for students.[2] Japan is not alone in beating the United States at this game. Nearly every Western European nation walks or uses bicycles considerably more than the United States does. Even our Canadian neighbors, culturally similar to us in many respects and facing a similarly sprawling landscape, manage to use bicycles for work-related trips three times as frequently as we do.[3] Cities that have improved walkability and encouraged foot and bicycle commuting have produced declines in obesity.[4]

Yet, for the last eighty years, we Americans have relentlessly worked to make our landscape less walkable. We build for ourselves unusually large homes on unusually large lots, and we prefer them to be freestanding, single-family homes surrounded by ornamental lawns.[5] To service our sparsely developed suburban landscapes, we build wide streets connected by enormous limited-access highways. In Japan, standard buildable lots are approximately one-twentieth of an acre; the standard for American suburbs is closer to three-fourths of an acre. Even the cores of our cities

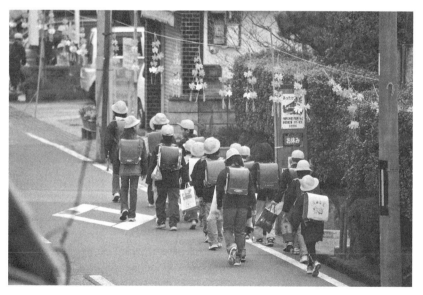

Japanese law dictates that schools in non-rural areas be within a walkable distance for children, and as a result, Japanese children walk to school more than anywhere else. Not surprisingly, Japan has among the world's lowest incidence of childhood obesity. *Colleen Miniuk Sperry/Alamy Stock Photo*

are substantially more sprawling than are the cores of cities in Europe and Asia. Within the city limits of Philadelphia and Washington, for example, the population density is roughly 10,000 people per square mile—sparse enough for many city residents to drive private cars from destination to destination. The core of Shanghai, by contrast, has a population density of over 250,000 people per square mile. Private automobile transport is thus almost unthinkable.

Our thinly populated cities are a marked departure from European cities of today, and even more so of a century ago. Nineteenth-century London, for example, was the largest city in the world and yet was mostly packed into a tight urban cluster about five miles across. Almost no place in the city was more than a two-hour walk from anyplace else. Other European cities, such as Vienna, Berlin, Amsterdam, and Budapest, were even smaller. The cores of these cities were populated at densities of 75,000 people per square mile: roughly the density of America's densest urban neighborhoods today in Manhattan. Residences, stores, workshops, churches, and schools were all built adjacent to each other. Kenneth Jackson, a historian

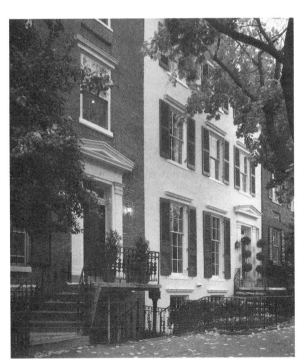

Traditional cities are more compact than post-war suburbs, making them far more walkable. These row houses are in the Georgetown neighborhood of Washington, DC. *Carol M. Highsmith Archive, Library of Congress, Prints and Manuscripts Division*

of American suburbia, estimated that in 1885 less than one worker in fifty walked more than one mile to work.[6] And the wealthy were no different, grabbing lots at the innermost precincts of these cities so they could be closer to banks, royalty, government offices, and other centers of power and commerce. Land on the outskirts of a city tended to be populated by those people lower on the social scale, such as workingmen, guildsmen, and seamen.

Early suburbs, when they did form, were governed by the same logic of foot travel. Rather than sprawl miles from transportation hubs, they tended to be built on a tight village model, with homes and businesses clustered around a village green. Early US suburbs such as Cambridge, Brooklyn Heights, and Greenwich Village were more sylvan and quiet but hardly pastoral. Homes were built on small lots; streets were narrow; and stores, businesses, and homes were intermixed. People may have appreciated privacy and sunlight, but the limits of shoe leather and fatigue dictated that people continued to live close to each other and to their most common destinations.

The explosive growth of the private automobile changed everything. Henry Ford's brilliant industrial coup in the first decades of the twentieth century allowed Americans unparalleled access to the open road. As the price of a Model T dropped to an incredible $290 by 1924 ($4,000 in 2018 dollars), it became pervasive. By 1926, the United States was building 85 percent of the world's cars, and Michigan alone counted more cars than Great Britain and Ireland.[7] By 1940, when one in five Americans owned a private car, only one in twenty-two Frenchmen could make that claim, and only one in fifty-four Germans.[8] Such broad ownership of private cars, when coupled with an unprecedented bout of road-building, wholly changed the landscape of America's built environment. With the passage of the Federal-Aid Highway Act of 1956, which created 42,000 miles of limited-access roadways, Americans' entire perception of time and distance was reconfigured. Traveling sixty-five miles per hour had become the norm. Henry Ford predicted, "The city is doomed."[9]

Developers responded to the automobile by building madly. In the 1920s, housing starts numbered 883,000 per year—double that of previous periods—and the vast majority of these starts were in new edge neighborhoods and suburbs that ringed major cities.[10] During this time, suburbs of major cities grew twice as fast as core neighborhoods. However, such growth was predicated on longer commutes by streetcar, bus, or

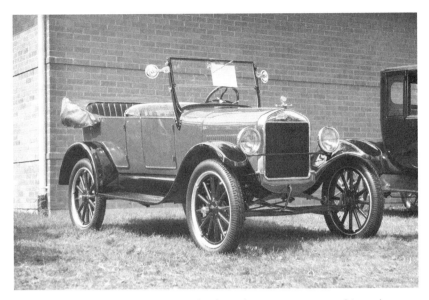

The famed Ford Model T; the vehicle that brought private car ownership to the masses. By 1926, the United States was selling 85 percent of the world's private cars. *Dreamstime Images*

automobile. Walking, first to work, and later to shopping and recreation, began to decline.

Building accelerated sharply after the war when returning GIs, flush with cheap loans, new wives, and newer babies, impelled private developers to put up 114,000 single-family homes in 1944, 937,000 in 1946, and an incredible 1,692,000 in 1950. Sales of suburban accouterments followed suit: lawnmower sales went from 42,000 in 1940 to over a million a decade later, and home freezer sales grew at the same pace.[11] With innovations in building techniques, such as William and Alfred Levitt's assembly-line operation to put up 34,000 houses in just a few years in their "Levittowns" outside of New York and Philadelphia, suburbia became affordable to all but the poorest.[12] By 1960, for the first time in the history of the country, American cities were actually shrinking. That year's census showed that fourteen of the nation's fifteen largest cities had actually lost population over the previous decade. (The sole exception was Los Angeles.) Political scientist Theodore White declared the threshold the "passage of the crest of the great city."[13] The new suburbs were poised to overtake their urban antecedents.

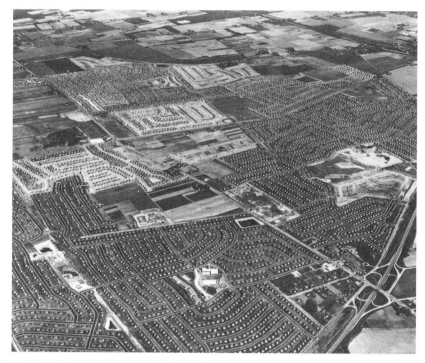

The original Levittown on Long Island. The two-bedroom houses could be purchased for $7,000, but owners gave up the walkable lives they had known in the city. *King Rose Archives/Global Image Works*

Suburban development was notably dominated by single-family, fully detached homes built at very low density. Virtually all houses were set back from the street, sometimes greatly so. Chevy Chase, Maryland, for example, an early first-ring suburb, required a twenty-five-foot setback for all homes. Streets were also far wider than traffic volume might dictate, with eighty feet being standard in Garden City, Long Island, versus a mere sixty-feet for midtown Manhattan. Many suburbs had minimum lot sizes of an acre or more; several towns in Northern Westchester and the northern Lakeshore suburbs in Illinois had five-acre minimums. Moreover, one-story houses built in ranch or bungalow styles were unusually popular, forcing population density even lower. The builders of Park Forest, Illinois, boasted that they were designing a development in which nearly 90 percent of the land would have no buildings, traditional blocks would disappear, and the "old-time downtown district" would be "nonexistent."[14]

Such ultra-low density presaged the development of second- and third-ring suburbs, the so-called "edge-city" and "exurb" developments of the 1970s. These developments tended to go beyond the end of commuter rail lines, forcing residents to drive many miles just to get to the last railroad stop, or (more likely) to forgo mass transit altogether and drive directly to work. Coatesville, Pennsylvania, was seventeen miles past the end of Philadelphia's suburban Paoli/Thorndale line, and the new developments in west Los Angeles—Bel Air, Palos Verdes Hills, and Rolling Hills—were as far west of the center city as Pasadena was to the east. The greatest exurban destination, Fairfield County, Connecticut, was in another state entirely. The most desired towns there—Reading, Darien, Westport, and Fairfield—were all at least sixty miles from midtown Manhattan, yet the population of the county grew from 400,000 in 1940 to 800,000 in 1975.[15]

Such development provided many Americans with comfortable indoor living spaces but at the expense of livable and walkable outdoor space. Wolfgang Langewiesche, writing an early critique of the development, noted:

> Here is the worst thing the house-on-lot system does: It causes sprawl. Suppose there was a law requiring an inch of air space between all dishes in your cupboard, all clothes in your closets, all books on your shelves: Your stuff would push you clear out of your house. That is what we have done to ourselves and to each other, with those pretty front lawns and innocent-looking side yards. We have pushed each other outward until New York (the real city, not the political unit so called) is eighty miles long and forty miles broad; Chicago eighty miles by thirty; and Greater Los Angeles, almost a country.[16]

Denizens of these new communities lived in a netherworld that was neither city nor farm. They had eschewed urban density but hardly embraced the physicality and organicism of the countryside. In doing so, they had managed to create for themselves a land of near perfect unwalkability. One critic termed the new landscape "subtopia," a "monster that is devouring in its bulldozer jaws some three thousand acres of green countryside daily."[17]

Suburbs were designed to ease congestion, and as such, their architects tended to shun the sort of mixed-use development common to older cities. Whereas the urban landscape tended to cluster stores, apartments, churches, schools, and offices all in the same neighborhood, and sometimes even in the same block, suburban designers tended to separate these functions into single-use zones. Residential neighborhoods were all houses and shopping zones were all retail. Offices, if they existed at all, were clustered in suburban office parks built at the edge of the suburban zones. Civic buildings, such as town halls, police stations, libraries, and schools, were often clustered in a civic zone.

The design created quiet neighborhoods but demanded automobile transportation for virtually every function. To ease the demands of the automobile, most buildings were surrounded by enormous parking lots that could be entered only off of busy, unwalkable, primary arteries. Intersections tended to have rounded corners, making turning easier from the road, but made crossing more difficult for pedestrians. To the partners of one design firm trying to rectify these elements, the gestalt of suburbia was "enforced in the name of a single objective: making cars happy."[18]

Between 1950 and 1970, developers built 22,000 new suburban shopping centers, virtually all predicated on easy parking and seamless automobile access.[19] In sprawling Atlanta, Georgia, the average trip to a supermarket was five miles.[20] In the exquisitely expensive precincts of San Jose, California, the heart of the microchip industry, desperate homebuyers

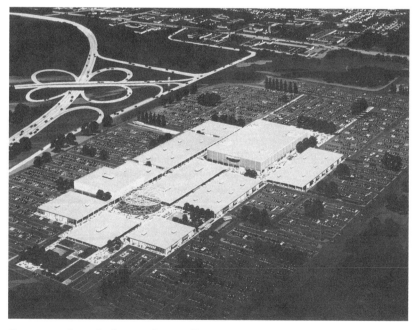

One reason that suburbanites don't walk is that most of their destinations are surrounded by enormous parking lots. This creates an unpleasant, dangerous, and hot approach for pedestrians. *The Everett Collection*

moved sixty miles away to Tracy, California, in an effort to find some suburban peace. One high-tech employee admitted, "I spent 2,048 hours working . . . 1,100 hours commuting . . . 608 with my family. I spent twice as much time driving as with my kids."[21]

But more than for commuters, the suburban landscape placed automotive demands on stay-home parents, usually mothers, who wound up making dozens of car trips weekly to soccer practice, school events, church meetings, Hebrew school, music lessons, play rehearsals, supermarkets and malls, restaurants and coffee shops, houses of friends, and, ironically, gyms and workout studios. So unwalkable were the suburbs that many well-intentioned suburbanites found themselves regularly driving themselves and their kids to places to ride a bike or take a walk. Suburban critics were well aware of the "drive to cross the street" phenomenon but driving to the walking path or bike path was equally common. Even as designers began to recognize the ills of the car-centered landscape, little could be done to undo decades of road design and land-use planning; poured cement could only be removed at enormous expense. Between 1984 and 2000, the average number of miles driven weekly by a stay-home suburban parent *doubled*.[22]

Lest I sound utterly despondent, the last two decades have witnessed the rise of the new urbanism, a movement among land-use planners to try to recreate some of the mixed-use walkability of urban neighborhoods in suburbs and edge cities. Some of these newly centered suburbs are retrofitted older suburbs; others, notably Celebration, Florida; Reston, Virginia; and Columbia, Maryland, are purpose-built.[23] Designers who adhere to new urban landscape design take as their model older, compact urban neighborhoods such as Georgetown, Alexandria, Greenwich Village, and Nantucket. They create dense, narrow streets with curbside parking and mixed-use buildings. Both residential and commercial spaces are built right up to the sidewalk with minimal side lots. Stores and offices are integrated into the streetscape, while major civic destinations are within a reasonable walk to the downtown. The designers at Duany Plater-Zyberk, a firm that personifies this sort of suburban design philosophy, point out that one of the reasons that people love Disneyworld is its recreation of an old-fashioned walkable main street. The irony is that for three-quarters of a century, we have done our best to destroy precisely these sorts of urban landscapes that we actually profess to love.

One thing we do know is that if we make it difficult for people to walk, they will not walk. People walk most not when they are avid lovers of hiking and the vigorous life but rather when walking is integrated into their daily living patterns. One study found a close association between the age of the neighborhood that people live in and how much they walk or bike; people living in neighborhoods built before 1947 walked or biked three times as frequently as people living in neighborhoods built after 1977.[24] People will gladly walk when it is the most reliable form of transportation to get to and from nearby stores, offices, subway stops, schools, and churches. Place these destinations in inaccessible lots surrounded by parking and accessible only by major arteries and most walking ceases. Those blessed with time (and money) can compensate for the loss of walking by joining private gyms, hiring personal trainers, and attending spin and aerobics classes, but for many Americans, these sorts of artificial fitness obligations are simply beyond their means. We have largely given up walking, and we are paying a steep price.

4

Changing Lives

Our environment has changed in more abstract ways. The pace of our days, the shape of our families, and the habits of our gender have all shifted substantially over the past half century, and these changes, too, affect our weight. We commute farther, work longer, eat more hurriedly, and sit—*plotz!*—more languorously. We eat many more of our meals alone and on the run. At the same time, many of the mealtime rituals that had bonded us and helped us maintain reasonable eating habits have eroded. On any commercial flight today, I can order my meal regular, vegetarian, Asian vegetarian, vegan, Kosher, Halal, low-sodium, and gluten-free. Such culinary autonomy reflects the individual ethos that Americans celebrate, but it also forces us each to reinvent our eating habits, losing many time-tested eating patterns that have helped us maintain a healthy weight.

HOME ECONOMICS

What could be less sexy than home economics? The discipline has largely dropped out of high school and college curricula, and even when retained, it has morphed into "human ecology" programs that focus on developmental psychology. However, for fifty years, home economics was a standard course of study for female high school students in the United States and for many college students as well. Whole departments of home economics were staffed with faculty who had earned PhDs in the field and published their research in peer-reviewed organs such as the *Journal of Home*

Economics. The curriculum produced generations of young American women who were facile in homemaking—knowing how to sew, clean, and cook. While few of us wish to see a return to such rigidly defined gender roles, I would argue that we do not fully appreciate the health effects of the demise of home economics.

Home economics has a founding mother in the person of Ellen Richards, a Vassar alum and MIT-trained chemist who was instrumental in establishing the American Home Economics Association in 1908. An instructor in sanitary chemistry at MIT, she, along with Marion Talbot at the University of Chicago's Department of Household Administration, worked to define home economics as a scientifically based approach to domesticity. Shopping, tailoring, cooking, and parenting could all be studied and optimized. If women were to spend their lives serving their households, they might as well do it well. Helen Campbell, another early home economics pioneer, dismissed the average housekeeper who talked about having "luck" with her sponge cake. "*Luck!*" wrote Campbell. "There is no such word in science, and to make a sponge cake is a scientific process."[1]

To some degree, home economics grew from the same impulse toward efficiency as the industrial engineering of Frank Gilbreth and Frederick Winslow Taylor in the early years of the twentieth century. These industrial consultants are remembered for their stopwatch motion studies of manufacturing processes; subjecting domestic tasks to similar efficiency studies was only one step behind. Gilbreth, best remembered as the freakishly compulsive father in *Cheaper by the Dozen*, encouraged his wife, Lillian Gilbreth, to apply their efficiency models to the household. Her son, Frank Jr., wrote years later that "every washing machine, kitchen stove, and refrigerator that rolls off the assembly lines today bears the imprint of her research."[2]

By 1916, nearly 18,000 college students were enrolled in home economics courses, and 26 percent of high schools offered courses. In 1923, the US Department of Agriculture established the Bureau of Home Economics, which was closely allied with women's organizations throughout the nation. Such groups as the League of Women Voters, the General Federation of Women's Clubs, the PTA, and the Woman's Christian Temperance Union worked to advise the new bureau, which was chartered to "study the relative utility and economy of agricultural products for food, clothing, and other uses in the home."[3] By 1939, 72 percent of high schools offered home economics courses, and nearly half of all high school girls took a home economics class in any given year.[4]

The impulse toward home economics was varied, ranging from pride of efficacy to national fortitude. For women who prided themselves on their domestic skills, the profession validated the seriousness with which they took their domestic charge. One home economist, who proudly bore the moniker of "housewife," wrote, "Ours is a true profession, ancient, honorable, and unique."[5] Others saw domesticity, particularly cooking, as the first line of defense against national dissolution. Home economics raised the efficiency of the American household and pushed women to cook more nutritiously while spending less money. Various studies of home economic students showed that they cooked more protein and fewer carbohydrates, all while spending less of the household budget on groceries than their

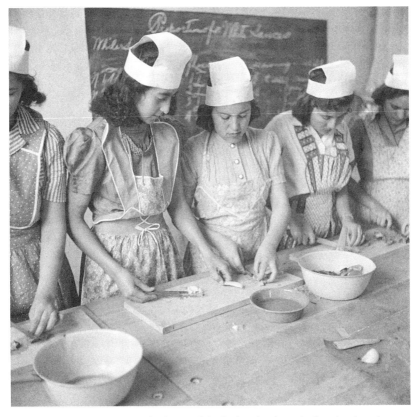

Home economics was a standard part of the high school curriculum for American girls until the late 1960s. Its removal from the curriculum has produced a generation of Americans who lack basic cooking skills and, thus, tend to eat more prepared foods and frequent restaurants. *Getty Images*

untrained peers.[6] Other, similar, studies showed lower rates of food spoilage and malnutrition in homes run by home economics graduates. One school superintendent advocated for the curriculum by defending its intellectual rigor. He wrote that home economics, "provides the content for the applications of scientific principles more thoroughly than does any other subject of study."[7] More colloquially, one proud grandmother bragged, "You can tell that my daughter had the vocational home economics course from the way her house looks and how healthy her children are!"[8]

Home economics presupposed a strong gender bias, with virtually all proponents and teachers of the curriculum, and most its students, being female. In theory, this need not have been so, given the long history of male cooks, and high schools in the United States experimented with integrating boys into the classes. Some were successful, finding that boys appeared to be interested, particularly when taught in single-sex classes.[9] However, in general, home economics was aimed overwhelmingly at girls with the knowledge that the majority would soon marry and take near total responsibility for domestic tasks. The assumption was hardly specious. In the decade after World War II, over 70 percent of American women married within four years of high school graduation.[10] In light of this, home economics teachers began to view their work in an almost religious light, taking upon themselves the future of the American family, if not society itself. One zealous home economics teacher wrote that her goal was to, "help my pupils develop an unshakeable belief in the sanctity of the marriage vows and in the value of indestructible family ties."[11]

FEMINISM

The cult of domesticity intensified in the years after World War II. Returning servicemen sought a sort of hyper-normality after the disruption of combat. Their yen was toward home, (suburban) hearth, and family; traditional gender roles ascended accordingly. Women's incomes in the United States actually declined in the decades after the war, dropping from 64 percent of male earnings in 1955 to 58 percent in 1968.[12] Age of first marriage fell; family size increased; and women's attendance in graduate and professional programs stagnated.

However, all was not bliss. Some women felt constrained by their heavily determined roles: under-challenged and over-objectified. This frustration, given voice by early feminists such as Betty Friedan, Kate Millett,

Katha Pollitt, and (in France) Simone de Beauvoir, exploded in demands for change in the 1960s. "I, like other women, thought there was something wrong with me because I didn't have an orgasm waxing the kitchen floor," wrote Friedan, bored and unsatisfied in an unhappy marriage in the New York suburbs.[13] Mainstream feminists, along with progressive government leaders, demanded a shift in gender roles, facilitated by accessible childcare, supportive men, equal pay laws, and—the Holy Grail—the hotly pursued Equal Rights Amendment (ERA) to the United States Constitution. Feminist political pioneers, such as Bella Abzug and Shirley Chisholm in Congress, Eleanor Holmes Norton of the Commission on Human Rights, and Bess Myerson of the New York City Department of Consumer Affairs, pushed for stricter enforcement of workplace equality and greater support for women's concerns. Such mainstream feminists sought a retention of existing societal structures but with a shift toward gender equality. One feminist protester in the late 1960s explained, "I keep telling my husband that either his ideas or mine will have to change, and . . . I get more and more convinced that it's going to have to be him."[14]

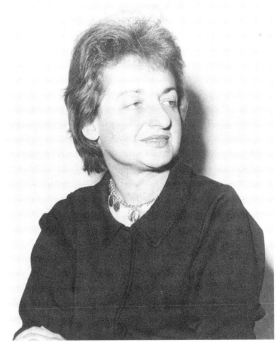

Betty Friedan became one of the leading voices of the modern feminist movement in the early 1960s when she expressed dissatisfaction with her life as a housewife. *King Rose Archives/Global Image Works*

Radical feminists, led by the fiery rhetoric of French philosopher Simone de Beauvoir, demanded more. For this group, essential structures needed to evolve or be discarded entirely. Marriage was suspect; even heterosexual relationships and the maternal drive were viewed skeptically. De Beauvoir conditioned the self-actualization of women on discarding the family itself, declaring, "As long as the family and the myth of the family and the myth of maternity and the maternal instinct are not destroyed, women will still be oppressed."[15] When asked what would replace the family as the basis of communal life, her reply was anything but sympathetic: "After all," she noted, "the American slaves didn't ask themselves what was going to happen to the American economy when they won their freedom."[16]

Other radical feminists of the late 1960s and early 1970s agreed, although their degree of man-hating varied. Kate Millett's 1970 feminist diatribe, *Sexual Politics*, echoed de Beauvoir's call for radically reimagining the essential nature of gender. Even her thesis advisor admitted, "Reading the book is like sitting with your testicles in a nutcracker."[17] The women of W.I.T.C.H. (Women's International Terrorist Conspiracy from Hell), Redstockings, and the New York Radical Women collective took their fight to corporate workplaces and attempted to change workplace norms.[18] In a departure, one thoughtful political science graduate student, a member of *fem lib* [sic], sounded not quite angry so much as inquisitive—willing to ponder the unknowable next chapter in gender relations and societal structures. "What does it mean?" she wrote.

> To me, liberation means a loosening-up of attitudes, a determination to be open-minded, a refusal to indulge in labels and categories. It means the freedom to explore new approaches to work, marriage, fatherhood, and motherhood. I am in *fem lib* because I want to destroy stereotypes. If you ask me what I choose to replace the old stereotypes with, I cannot give you an answer because I honestly don't know them. But that is the whole point. I prefer open-endedness to the deceptive security of conforming to settled, socially defined roles.[19]

Such revolutionary sentiment inspired a backlash, and millions of women not only refrained from joining the movement but deepened their commitment to traditional roles and the family. Phyllis Schlafly, a Republican operative who had opposed Richard Nixon at the 1960 Republican Convention for being overly liberal, became the leading voice of opposition to the Equal Rights Amendment in the 1970s, and she was instrumental in defeating it.[20] Many ardently Christian women saw the drive toward liberation in direct contradiction of Biblical morals. One wrote, "A Christian woman puts things in the proper perspective, namely: 1) God and the Bible; 2) husband; 3) children; 4) herself." Another woman, active in the Moral Majority political organization, concurred: "I have served my family twenty-five years, and I'll do it 'till the day I die, and you humanists will never change us! A true Christian husband appreciates an unselfish, devoted wife who makes *him* her life. He would *never* leave her. Only secular men do that!"[21]

Other, secular women were no less repulsed by the shift afoot. These women, content in their marriages and domesticity, questioned the need for such radical change. Celebrating their attractiveness and sexuality, many admitted to enjoying the dance of flirtation, the attention of men. "I love the idea of looking delectable and having men whistle at me," admitted one professional woman in Los Angeles.[22] The New York Pussycat League, a group of women dedicated to traditional women's sexual roles, adopted as their mantra, "The lamb chop is mightier than the karate chop."[23]

It is worth noting that the feminist revolution was largely the purview of white, middle-class women who resented the domestic constraints in which they were living in the 1960s. Many women had always worked, either by choice or necessity, and African American author Toni Morrison summed up black women's feelings toward women's liberation as "distrust" for what was basically a "family quarrel between white women and white men."[24] Nevertheless, the movement had a profound effect on women's roles in American life. From 1968 to 1972, the women's share of delegates at the Democratic National Convention grew from 13 percent to 40, and at the Republican Convention, from 17 to 29. Starting in the early 1970s, female enrollment in medical and law schools grew dramatically, reaching parity with men by the year 2000. Women claimed only one seat in the US Senate in 1970; by 2016, they claimed twenty. By almost any measure, the presence of women in virtually all walks of American professional life grew dramatically starting in 1970, despite the failure of the passage of the ERA.

CHANGING FAMILIES

Families, too, changed rapidly in the 1970s. Divorce rates soared. Between 1950 and 1993, the portion of children in the United States being raised by two married parents at home dropped from 77 to 55 percent. The portion of poor children raised by two married parents dropped to 35 percent. Out-of-wedlock births rose from 5 to 26 percent. Single-person households grew from 12 to 27 percent. Adolescent suicide doubled.[25]

Children raised in single-parent households did significantly worse along nearly all axes of accomplishment. After a divorce, their grades declined and their truancy rose. Behaviors that were correlated with long-term failure—early pregnancy, alcohol and drug use, dropping out of school—all rose. At the most basic level, poverty rose. Men paying child-support (when they could be induced to pay child support) transferred, on average, $3,000 per year to their children. By contrast, married men tended to transfer nearly all of their income to their household.[26]

Girls growing up in divorced families tended to become sexually active earlier. One study showed that female adolescent clients, upon meeting with a male social worker, tended to choose different seating arrangements upon entering the office. Daughters of married couples tended to sit across from the social worker to make direct eye contact; daughters of divorce tended to sit next to the social worker and adopt more suggestive poses.[27] That is, divorce disrupted adolescent sexual boundaries, impelling girls into more sexualized interactions with the adults in their lives.

Boys, too, were affected by divorce, albeit in different ways. Oddly, sons of divorce were more likely to adopt more traditional views of gender, and they were less able to construct socially egalitarian partnerships with future girlfriends and wives. Margaret Mead, a noted anthropologist, commented on precisely this when she wrote, in 1949, that in many cultures, "men's sureness of their sex role is tied up with their right, or ability, to practice some activity that women are not allowed to practice."[28] Boys raised in cultures with more intensive paternal investment tended to view men and women as more equal partners and were "more willing to share with women broad social power and authority," in the words of sociologist David Popenoe.[29]

When coupled with a greater number of working women, divorce and single-parenthood undermined traditional eating habits. Family dinners became far more difficult to sustain when the person previously responsible for preparing meals worked fulltime. Full-time work and divorce (and single parenthood) placed time and financial pressures on family units wherein rituals were marginalized, or dispensed with altogether. Both adults and children ate out more or ate prepared meals at home on their own. As we will see in coming sections, these changes in habits made sense given the time and financial pressures being placed on households but ultimately undermined patterns that had facilitated healthy eating habits.

CHANGES IN WORK AND CHANGING PLAY

Suburbanization meant less walking, but so too did changes in the workplace and changes in leisure. As the American economy evolved from the industrial orientation that had grounded it for a century, many jobs became more sedentary. The new cogitative economy demanded a huge class of workers that Robert Reich, Secretary of Labor under President Bill Clinton, called *symbol analysts*—that is, people who made a living by consuming, analyzing, manipulating, and producing information.[30] Graphic designers, computer programmers, journalists, attorneys, professors, statisticians, systems engineers, clerks, human resources professionals, and administrators of all types made their livings by spending large portions of their day sitting at a desk in front of a computer terminal. Professions that had once been more physically active—journalism, for example—were often being done over a phone or the internet.

Moreover, Americans were spending more time at work. The average workweek for salaried professionals grew to over fifty hours by 2010, with over a quarter of all white-collar workers reported working more.[31] When coupled with ever-lengthening commutes, the typical college-educated American in the labor force practically lived in a chair. Two exercise physiologists wrote in 1980: "When five o'clock rolls around, America becomes a virtual game of musical chairs. People rush from their professional sitting spots to other seats—at bars, at kitchen tables, and on assorted means of transportation."[32]

When people rushed home, they sat in their easy chairs to read, sip cocktails, chat with friends and spouses, and nap. However, starting in the early 1950s, what they did increasingly in their easy chairs was watch television.

Television viewing rose exponentially through the 1950s and 1960s, such that by 1975, the average American watched over four hours of television daily. Americans spent more time watching television than they spent doing nearly anything else, save sleeping and working. American children spent much more time watching television than doing homework, and as they watched more television, they spent less time playing outside. Not surprisingly, the rise of television viewing dovetailed nearly perfectly with the rise of childhood obesity.[33]

Adult television viewing correlated with obesity as well. Studies in the 1980s showed that adult women who watched more than three hours of television per day were twice as likely to be obese as women who watched less.[34] All people who watched more television tended to eat; children ate more junk food, and adults generally ate more. Television watching not only slowed metabolism, but it also seemed to undermine self-restraint. People ate more while they watched, and then they continued to eat more once they turned the set off. Television watching seemed to transform viewers into a semi-zombie state, where their ability to control their appetites, or even be aware of their eating, was squashed. That is, any sedentary activity was obviously insalubrious, but television watching seemed to be uniquely insalubrious relative to other sedentary activities such as chatting, reading, or working.[35]

Researchers were not exactly sure why this was so. Television viewers, particularly children, were subjected to a blitz of food commercials. Snack food, fast food, beer, and soda companies all advertised heavily on television. It was possible that the images of people eating and drinking spurred appetites. Or it was possible that the nature of television viewing brought on a certain passivity associated with mindless eating. Possibly, too, people watched television together and tended to eat socially while watching.

An alternative theory was that excessive television viewing did not so much cause obesity as indicate certain class and character traits otherwise associated with obesity. More highly educated people, who also tended to be wealthier, watched less television, and they also tended to eat less. Television may thus have simply signaled education and class, which themselves were the true determinants of obesity. Or perhaps excessive television viewing may have been associated with depression and anxiety disorders in which excessive eating was again implicated.

Many researchers suspected that for children, television viewing specifically displaced more physically active pastimes. Kids did not watch television in place of attending school, but they did watch television in place of playing more actively, such as engaging in sports or riding their bikes. The hours spent watching television in the afternoons were displacing the few hours of physical activity that kids had previously gotten between sitting in school and being driven home.

Whatever the explanation, television was strongly correlated with *snacking*, which became commonplace in the United States in the 1970s. The snacking culture, exacerbated by chaotic households, unpredictable mealtimes, and excessive television watching, was at direct odds with one of the few Western countries that was doing a better job keeping its weight down by the early 2000s. France, famously chic and slim, was growing fatter, but at a slower rate than was Germany, the United Kingdom, and the United States. French slimness was enigmatic, given the relatively high fat content of the French diet and the emphasis on heavy, traditional sauces, but observers pointed out that if one looked closely at *how* the French were eating, rather than at *what* the French were eating, one might find clues to their ability to ward off obesity.

The French simply refused to snack. Eating in France remained, as had once been true in the United States, a social pastime: an activity preserved nearly exclusively for defined mealtimes with family and friends. French public schools served hot lunches for all children every day, and kids were expected to partake. By 2000, nearly 90 percent of all French children were eating dinner each night at home with their families every night, as opposed to about 40 percent of American children. Although French restaurants were famous throughout the world, the French actually spent a substantially lower portion of their food budget eating out than did Americans. French meals were slower (typically one hour for dinner), multi-course, more leisurely, and more social. French schoolchildren were allocated a full thirty minutes to eat their lunch while in school, versus the twenty minutes that frantic American school systems allowed kids. And while the French had a long established snack time for children right after school (*le gouter*), the snack time was sharply delineated: one modest piece of chocolate cake, and the kitchen was closed until dinner. Karen Le Billon, a Canadian living in France, marveled at French eating norms:

> This effect is heightened by the rules concerning *how* the French eat. Food is never eaten standing up, or in the car, or on the go. Food is not eaten anywhere, in fact, but at the table. And food is only served when *everyone* is at the table. "*A table!*" is a summons that brings most French children running. Everyone waits for everyone else to be served, and for the ritual "*Bon appétit!*" to be said before beginning the meal. As children almost always eat with their parents, these habits sink in early.[36]

Le Billon's observations about French eating norms dovetail with anthropological and paleontological insights into human eating patterns. Humans are uniquely social eaters. Other animals eat in parallel; that is, they sit next to each other while eating their own food. Only human beings deliberately prepare and share food. The *hearth*, that great symbol of the communal meal, dates from hundreds of thousands of years ago. Ancient fire pits have been found with knife-marked animal bones from large animals that were almost certainly shared.[37] Meal-sharing probably began in response to group-hunting: the strategy used when smaller animals bring down a larger one. However, whereas other animals hunt in packs (wolves, sharks, even ants), only humans prepare their meal together. That is, *cooking* is uniquely human, and it seems to have co-evolved with our communal norms. To be human is to be social, and to be social is to dine together. When we depart too far from these ancient norms, we seem to damage many of the delicate feedback systems that govern our appetites and our satiety.

Yet in today's America, we have departed substantially from our historic culinary norms. An entire generation has come of age that lacks basic cooking skills. In response, we eat out; we eat take-out; we eat fast; and we eat alone. Long commutes and longer working hours only make the trend worse.

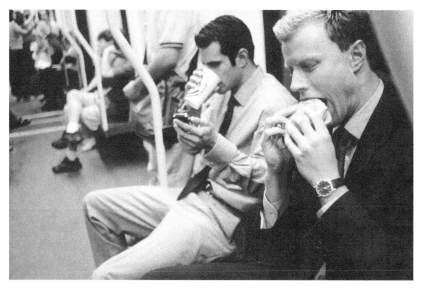

Breakdown in traditional eating norms has been exacerbated by hectic schedules and long commutes. These young men are eating on a subway train: a breach of etiquette that would have been unthinkable even a generation ago. *age fotostock/ Alamy Stock Photo*

Our lives have changed dramatically in a very short period of time. In the space of just a few generations, we have integrated into our lives cars, smartphones, television (and YouTube), the information economy, long-distance relationships, take-out food, information-based work, central heating, and solitary living. Such changes have brought enormous benefits to billions, including broad distribution of literacy, modern medical care, social mobility, gender equality, and physical safety. However, such changes have also played havoc with our eating habits. Primitive forces that have traditionally governed how we prepared and consumed food have rapidly been broken down. The symbol of the hearth for the millennial generation is not the dinner table but the coffee table, over which today's twenty-something leans into a carton of take-out Chinese food, eating alone while watching television. It's a far cry from the hearth of yesteryear.

5

Changing Food/Changing Meals

PROCESSED FOOD

Our lives and our habitats have changed dramatically, and so too has our food. Through most of history, we hunted, dug, collected, and grew almost everything that we put into our mouths. Although we learned to cook our food nearly 100,000 years ago—in a sense beginning the digestion process outside of our bodies—we did little else to our food until about 4,000 years ago when we learned to mill grains to increase the surface area of the proteins within and reduce absorption time. There we rested for millennia, still shooting game, picking and growing vegetables, baking whole-grain breads, and (a special treat!) preserving fruits for winter by cooking them with sugar into jams and preserves or air-drying them. If your grandmother had met her great-great-great-grandmother, they could have comfortably shared recipes and kitchen tips.

In the past century, however, the ways we manipulate, prepare, and store foodstuffs have changed dramatically. Through deep-freezing, precooking, microwaving, assembling, hydrogenating, and chemically preserving food, we have created an environment where manipulated foods now dominate our diets. We have stripped out much of the fiber and bran in our carbohydrates, ground up and reconstituted our meats with extra salt and sugar, deep-frozen our vegetables, and precooked our dinners to the point that most of our food, in the words of food-guru Michael Pollan, "is no longer, strictly speaking, food at all."[1] Much of our food is now the product of processes that appear more industrial than agricultural, from monocultured agro-farms to poultry "processing" plants to artificial and "natural" flavors to chemical additives. What results is a highly processed, hyper-palatable, super-cheap food-like stuff that requires little chewing and less cleanup. It is no wonder that Pollan begins one of his celebrated polemics with a simple mantra: "Eat food. Not too much. Mostly plants."[2]

To some degree, we can trace our modern yen toward processing our food to the mid-nineteenth century with Cyrus McCormick's reaper and the first freight rail cars. These two developments allowed us to *commodify* the grains produced on America's farms, allowing middlemen and wholesalers to mill, sort, grade, and ship it to large feedlots and grain silos in rail hubs.[3] By 1870, in a parallel industrial process, meatpackers Gustavus Swift and Philip Armour had mastered the art of canning meats, preserving them for faraway customers who could store the goods in their pantries for months. Fish and fruit canning started soon after, with salmon coming by rail from California and fruit by steamer from the Caribbean and Central America.[4]

A second revolution began in 1925 when Clarence Birdseye patented his process for deep-freezing food. Birdseye had worked as a missionary in Labrador, Canada, in 1912 and had noticed that food frozen below a certain temperature remained palatable and unspoiled months later. Envisioning a vast change to the American diet, he industrialized the process with newly developed commercial deep freezers. By 1945, he was freezing 600,000 pounds of fresh vegetables a year and selling them to retail customers for $200 million.[5] American homemakers took rapidly to the convenience of frozen food, filling their homes with newly available deep freezers that could keep foods at temperatures below twenty degrees for months on end. Women's magazines pushed the trend, warning housewives in 1945, "So, if you don't want to be frozen out of the conversation, you'd better bone up."[6] *House Beautiful*, along with other women's magazines, published a primer on freezing in the immediate post-war years, celebrating the process's many benefits: "Quick freezing will abolish seasons . . . simplify meal preparations . . . enable you to serve famous dishes by famous chefs from famous restaurants . . . allow you to serve rare delicacies . . . banish the monotony of leftovers."[7]

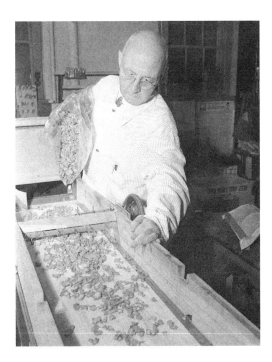

Clarence Birdseye
Getty Images

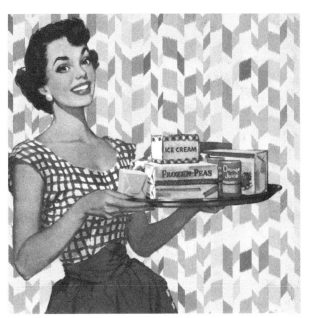

Clarence Birdseye
ushered in the
modern age of
prepared foods
when he started
marketing frozen
vegetables and
meats in 1925.
Twenty years later,
he was selling
600,000 pounds of
frozen vegetables
a year.

Frozen foods rapidly attracted a broad following. The advantages to farmers, ranchers, slaughterers, and distributors were obvious: Frozen foods could be distributed and sold year-round rather than simply in season, and they could be held in inventory for months rather than days. Frozen foods held at least some of their flavor, and when packed with sugar and salt, they could be made (sometimes) as palatable as the original. Whole new industries sprang up: refrigerated rail cars and trucks, refrigerator cases at grocery stores, frozen storerooms at wholesalers and restaurants. Whole new "all-frozen" stores sprang up, selling only frozen foodstuffs, sometimes with famous provenances. One store in suburban Chicago specialized in foods from a particularly prominent Chicago Italian restaurant.[8] Refrigerator companies offered to fully refrigerate grocery stores and brand them for a modest investment: essentially an early form of franchising.[9] Cooking columnists extolled the advantages of the "package to plate—nonstop!" revolution, pointing out the "quick-meal magic" that could be produced using canned and frozen foods, "custom packaged, to match the perfection of blue-sky June days."[10] One breathless reporter told of industry plans to grow the frozen food market to $11 billion annually—about two-thirds of all food bought and sold in the United States in a given year.[11] When coupled with the growth of canning and drying, frozen food impelled revolutionary change across America's kitchens through the 1950s and 1960s.

But beyond freezing, American food has become substantially more *processed* in the past century, in the sense that raw foodstuffs are now substantially manipulated and transformed before we begin to cook with them, much less actually eat them. The most basic way we process food is in milling grain—grinding and husking raw grain kernels into cracked, rolled, mealed, and ground products. We have milled grain for millennia, but in the past hundred years, we have taken to removing progressively more of the nutritive husks and skins of the grain kernels: the parts that we now collectively call bran. The whole-wheat flours, grits, rolled oats, and whole-grain cereals of our grandparents have been transformed into white goods—instant oatmeal, bleached flour, white rice, for example. Along the way, we have removed about 98 percent of all of the grain beyond the germ and along with it all of the fiber and the preponderance of nutrients.[12]

Bleached flour has been present in our diet for a century, but in the post-war years, food companies increased their manipulation of foodstuffs to make them more convenient and palatable but less nutritious. Canned fruits with peels removed; meats with skins gone; vegetables that had been bleached and then canned or frozen with salt and sugar all appealed to the changing American diet. Along the way, the ratio of calories to nutrients grew, such that by the 1950s, Americans were suffering from a malady specific to modern food preparation: they were "overfed and undernourished."[13] As supermarkets shelves became crowded with thousands of new prepared products, Americans became less aware of what they were actually putting in their bodies. Ingredient labels ran for paragraphs and included mysterious hydrogenated and processed oils along with elusive natural and artificial flavors and colors. Americans ate more meals that were loaded with fat, sugar, and salt, all while being stripped of fiber, skins, pits, bones, peels, and pith. Canned meals, such as Chef Boyardee products with precooked pastas, meats, and sauces, are all ready to heat on a stovetop and have dominated the American diet, along with cake and Jell-O mixes, television dinners, and every sort of premixed sauce and precut starch. Glenna Matthews, a historian of American domesticity, defines the 1950s as the "nadir" of American cookery, the "heyday of prepared foods and cream of mushroom soup cuisine," in which canned fruit, potato chips, marshmallows, and canned fish became staple ingredients of the American kitchen.[14]

Two additional machines added to the deskilling of the American cook: the pressure cooker, which gained popularity in the years following World War II, and the microwave oven, which gained acceptance in American kitchens in the 1970s.[15] Both tools could be used to expand a home cook's range while easing food preparation, and both shortened cooking times. Pressure cookers were marketed as the busy housewife's dream, allowing her to prepare "the same lusty dish" she "once hovered over . . . in fifteen to twenty minutes."[16] In a world of mechanization and modernity, fast-food preparation began to seem not merely convenient but meritorious. Processed food was scientific food: consistent, hyper-palatable, and long-lasting. Expanding numbers of food items, from frozen peas to canned meats to dried cereals, now had shelf lives of weeks or months. Foodstuffs that actually spoiled began to seem primitive, even unhealthy. Food that could harbor bacteria on the shelf was food that could harbor bacteria in the body. And bacteria, everybody knew by the 1950s, were the enemy of hygiene and health.[17]

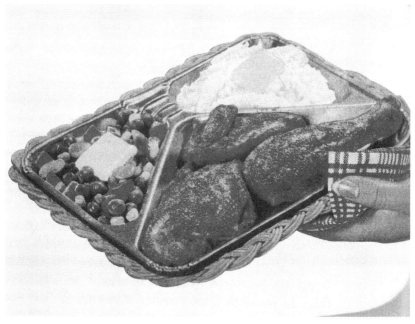

Birdseye's process lead to the frozen prepared dinner, which came to be known as TV dinners after many Americans began eating them off of trays while watching television in the 1950s. Although convenient, the product accelerated the decline of the family meal. *Getty Images*

Perhaps most foreboding in this trend was the increasing amount of sugar that food manufacturers pumped into their products. The American appetite for sugar seemed to be insatiable, and with sugar prices ever declining, the choice to infuse previously unsweetened products with sugar was an easy one. Products that had never before included sugar did so now. Ketchup, rice, vegetables of all sorts, tomato sauce, chicken and meat dishes, yogurt, cottage cheese, milk (in the form of the explosively popular chocolate and strawberry milk that appeared on refrigerator shelves in the 1960s), and even fish filets were now tinged with sugar. Perhaps the greatest offenders were the breakfast cereal manufacturers, who found that by sugar-coating old products—cornflakes, crisped rice, rolled oats—they could now sell much, much more of the stuff. The trend toward hyper-sweetened cereal reached its height (or its low) in the 1970s with such favorites as Froot Loops, Count Chocula, Quisp, Quake, and Lucky Charms—the last of which was suffused with multicolored marshmallows.

The public interest group Science in the Public Interest found its own favorite in Mr. Wonderfull's Surprize [sic]—a sugared nutritional horror show consisting of "little balls filled with a goo of sugar and saturated fat"—essentially mini-Twinkies in a bowl.[18]

FAST FOOD/HEDONIC FOOD

Fast food competed head-to-head with processed food in the post-war years, although its genesis can be traced back to the 1904 World's Fair in St. Louis, which is where Americans learned to eat hot dogs, soda, and ice-cream cones while walking around the fairgrounds. While Americans had long made sassafras tea and fruit juices at home, this Fair popularized the newly brewed Dr. Pepper, Hires' Root Beer, and Coca-Cola. Americans also learned to love the prototypes of popsicles at the fair—tubes of frozen lemonade that could be licked on the go—as well as Jell-O and cotton candy. When the Fair closed after seven months, it had "changed how the Western world ate and snacked," in the words of food historian Elizabeth Abbott.[19]

Short-order restaurants proliferated through the 1920s and 1930s, particularly in response to the growing popularity of the automobile. Roadside diners serving standard American meat-and-potato cuisine lined the nation's highways, and increasing numbers of businessmen chose to take their lunches at informal restaurants rather than walk home midday to eat in the kitchen. However, the fast-food restaurant—a uniquely American creation featuring utensil-free entrees built around the hamburger and various sorts of meat sandwiches—was not really invented until after World War II.

Richard and Maurice McDonald opened their drive-in hamburger place in San Bernardino, California, in 1940. Using multiple "car-hops"—waitresses who took orders and brought food to customers while they waited in their cars—the restaurant churned out cash and made the brothers rich within a few years. In 1948, looking to increase volume and revenue, the brothers jettisoned the car-hops and streamlined the menu to just a few items: hamburgers, soft drinks, and french fries. Food items were prepared on spec—that is, cooked before any customer had ordered them. The resulting process greatly increased throughput, even if it resulted in greater waste. When coupled with all disposable wrappers, cups, napkins, and utensils, the new McDonald's restaurant became the model for all subsequent fast food.

The new model was franchisable. The menu and process could be easily replicated by any enterprising entrepreneur who was willing to put up the capital for the kitchen and eating area. When coupled with contractual agreements to purchase supplies and raw ingredients from the corporate center, franchising allowed the rapid expansion of fast-food restaurants throughout the United States. Other chains quickly followed with similar preparation and consumption models, if not identical menus. Carl's, Wendy's, Burger King, Burger Chef, and Hot Shoppe Jr. all used assembly-line approaches to preparing and selling restaurant food in enormous volume at low prices through the 1960s and 1970s. The food was so cheap that restaurant meals became an affordable luxury for working-class families.[20]

Fast food was the perfect treat for tired families looking to sate everybody with minimal mess at low cost. The food—salted meats covered in sweet ketchup-based sauces, consumed with salted fried potatoes and Cokes—appealed to everybody. Later additions to the lineup, including fried chicken nuggets, breaded and fried fish fillets, fried chicken sandwiches, and multilayered cheeseburger creations, all leveraged the appeal

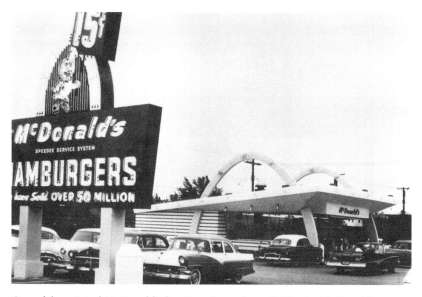

One of the original McDonald's locations in southern California. McDonald's and other fast-food chains largely displaced the old diners and Howard Johnson's restaurants throughout much of the country. They restricted their menus almost entirely to hamburger sandwiches, which could be eaten quickly and without utensils. *The Everett Collection*

of fatty meats mixed with salt and sugar and served on soft, sweet rolls. Fast-food restaurants were particularly adept at marketing the fare to kids, using toy giveaways and cartoon marketing figures to win over the younger generation. One survey found that more American kids could correctly identify Ronald McDonald than any other fictional character, save Santa Claus.[21]

By the year 2000, Americans were spending half of their food budget on meals eaten outside the house and consuming a third of their calories in restaurants. Many of these calories were eaten in the nation's 170,000 fast-food restaurants (including pizza places) where meals tended to be higher in fat and calories than meals prepared at home.[22] Serving sizes tended to grow at these restaurants, where restaurateurs found that they could sell more food at an additional profit by enlarging portions and "supersizing" meals. The size of a small Coke, for example, increased from six and a half ounces in the 1950s to sixteen ounces by 2000. Hamburgers, french fry servings, and desserts grew concomitantly. A typical fast-food dinner at the turn of the century clocked in at 2,000 calories—roughly a day's entire caloric requirement for an adult male. And the whole thing could be consumed in less than ten minutes.

Fast-food marketing succeeded. The strategy of speed, consistency, and ubiquity worked to habituate Americans to eating multiple meals weekly in the restaurants. The average American in 2000 consumed three hamburgers and four portions of french fries each week. Teenagers going to school near fast-food restaurants ate more of the food than teenagers with longer walks. One study in 2009 found that high school kids going to school within a half mile of a fast-food restaurant ate fewer vegetables, drank more soda, and were more likely to be overweight than their peers who had farther to walk.[23] Moreover, while the greater obesity may have reflected underlying demographics—fast-food chains tended to put restaurants in poorer neighborhoods, where residents were fatter to begin with—no such effect was found with smoking or other vices marketed to low-income groups.

Fast-food restaurants were not the only vendors moving food toward the "bliss point"—that point of optimum allure achieved through mixing fat, sugar, and salt. Restaurants throughout America were interested in getting customers to buy more food, to enjoy the food more, and to eat the food faster. Commercial chefs working in test kitchens have devised a variety of ways in which to lard seemingly innocuous base ingredients with large amounts of fat, sugar, and salt. Nachos, for example, the Americanized

Tex-Mex appetizer, starts with a base of fried corn tortillas upon which are layered cheese, guacamole, and sour cream, with salted beans or cured meats on top. Stuffed potato skins use a similar layered approach, as do (amazingly) most garden salads, in which the chips or potato skins are really just replaced with lettuce leaves and then layered again. The Cheesecake Factory's menu features Buffalo Blasts—"Chicken breast, cheese, and our spicy buffalo sauce, all stuffed in a spiced wrapper and fried until crisp. Served with celery sticks and blue cheese dressing."[24] The flour tortilla wrapper in that last dish is so absorbent in the deep-frying process that one food consultant calls it a "fat bomb."[25]

Cheese is a special culprit in these dishes. Cheap, fatty, salty, and tasty, it is now everywhere—drizzled on beans and soups, injected into eggs and crusts (the infamous "double-stuffed pizza"), and layered on meats, salads, and vegetables. American casual restaurants have embraced "cheesiness" as the optimal descriptor for all sorts of dishes that were never previously cheesy at all. Some Americans are surprised when they travel abroad and find that many cheese-laden dishes in the United States—pizzas, hamburgers, beans, salads, schnitzel—are, in fact, cheese-free in their original iterations.

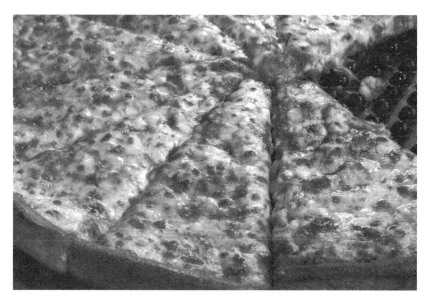

American foods have gotten fatter and larger. Pizzas are regularly touted as "extra cheesy." Some purveyors even inject cheese into the crust. *Ugur Anahtarci/Alamy Stock Photo*

There is no one culprit in America's obesity epidemic, and I hesitate to demonize McDonald's. Nonetheless, the fast-food industry, coupled with the sodas it frequently enters cobranding agreements with, bears a disproportionate share of the blame. The industry's hyper-palatable products, insidious youth-oriented marketing, low prices, and omnipresence have pushed fast-food spending to $110 billion annually. When coupled with declining kitchen skills, dwindling mealtime formalities, single-parent or dual-career households, and kinetic childhood scheduling, fast food has both enabled and responded to the deterioration of America's eating habits.

These restaurants have not only made cheap food palatable—really, unnaturally palatable to the point that our appetite control functions were never designed to resist—they have also created food that goes down remarkably quickly. Bones and skins are removed, vegetables and meats shredded, fibrous tissue cooked down until near mush. The chewy, crusty whole-grain breads of yesteryear have been replaced with Charmin-soft white breads; the fatty, fibrous meats are now boiled, ground, marinated, and tenderized to baby-food purees. Meat processing plants now subject chicken and beef cutlets to an injection treatment, in which a press with dozens of needles pushes into a slab of meat and injects it with marinades and tenderizers. One prominent turkey wholesaler labels its products "Butterball"—a perfect metaphor for this era of processed, flavored, fattened, and tenderized ingredients.

Perhaps the exemplar of this lab-tested sort of hyper-palatable, perfectly consumable, irresistible food is the Cinnabon brand cinnamon roll, found in malls, airports, and train stations across the country. The rolled buns are saturated with fat and coated in sugared syrup, and the wafting scents of cinnamon and freshly baked white bread set salivary glands awash. David Kessler describes the experience: "Then a series of flavors and textures unfold as I bite into the pillowy dough and taste the sweet, slippery filling and creamy frosting." A tasting partner comments, "It melts in your mouth. It disappears easily."[26]

Along with ramping up the tastiness of food, fast food and fast casual restaurants have increased standard portion sizes. Perhaps that last sentence is a misnomer, as one of the challenges that dieters face in the United States today is the lack of a standard portion size. Sodas now clock in at sixteen ounces (small), twenty-four ounces (medium), thirty-two ounces (large), and forty-eight ounces (supersize). Virtually all chain restaurants have inflated their standard serving size over the past generation. The typical meal of a burger, fries, and a Coke at McDonald's is now 1,100

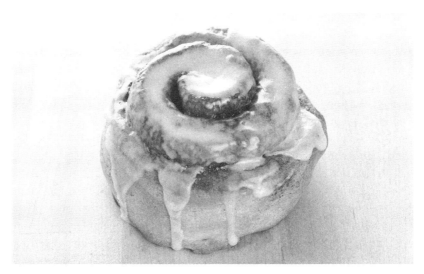

Cinnabon—the ultimate in hyper-palatable foods. Each serving packs in 880 calories. With their sweet, gooey doughiness and cinnamon aroma, they are irresistible to many people. *Brent Hofacker/Alamy Stock Photo*

calories, with supersizing bringing it to 1,400 with ninety-five grams (nineteen teaspoons) of sugar.[27] One food writer observed that "graphing the size of McDonald's largest burgers, from the Big Mac to the Double Quarter Pounder and the Triple Cheeseburger, is like watching America's appetite grow before your eyes."[28]

Inflated restaurant portions seem to be a particularly potent source of overeating, as diners have proven to be largely inept at estimating portion size. Fifty years of supersizing has recalibrated many Americans' idea of what constitutes a reasonable portion for an adult. Many nutritionists spend their first sessions with clients teaching them to subtract half, or even two-thirds, off of what the clients had previously thought of as a portion. Most Americans, who have not been through training, are lousy at estimating portion sizes. Multiple studies have demonstrated that eaters anchor their portions to what is served to them; that is, they assume that the served portion is reasonable, and they go from there. One study of college students served three groups of students meals for a week that were a) the same size as they estimated that they usually ate; b) 25 percent greater in size; and c) 50 percent greater in size. "No surprise," the authors wrote. "The groups served the most ate the most."[29]

More sobering is that most people rapidly adapt to larger portion sizes. A research team fed a group of study participants two meals a day for two successive eleven-day periods in a controlled setting. In the first period, the researchers served the participants normal-size portions. In the second eleven-day period, researchers served the participants portions that were 50 percent larger than normal. The researchers wanted to know if the subjects would revert to their normal eating habits during the second phase. They did not. The typical subject ate 423 calories more each day when served larger portions.[30] Other studies have served bottomless bowls of soup and enormous tubs of popcorn to subjects. The subjects eat and eat and eat, unaware of how much they have consumed, and they are often unaware that they have eaten more than usual. The commercial effects of this phenomenon are clear. One dessert at an Applebee's restaurant chain, the Blue Ribbon Brownie, has 1,600 calories, which is equal to a dessert for eight people. It's sold as a single portion.[31]

Portion sizes have grown, in part, because the raw ingredients are so cheap. American farms and slaughterhouses are today producing 3,700 calories per day for every American: too much for a grown man, and way

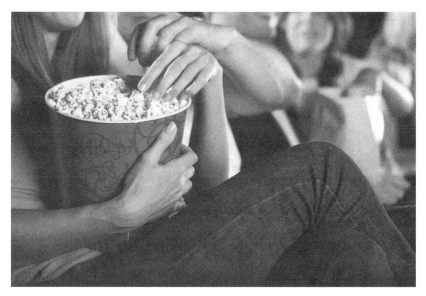

The "supersizing" of American restaurant portions has made it difficult for many Americans to estimate a reasonable portion. This popcorn is marketed as a single serving. *Kzenon/Alamy Stock Photo*

too much for a grown woman or child. Red meat, once a luxury for the middle-class, is now standard fare; non-vegetarian Americans consume nearly two pounds of it each week. Turkey and chicken are now so cheap that they are standard ingredients in the Food Stamps basket. Carbohydrates are practically free. A one-pound loaf of generic white bread, containing 3,600 calories, often retails for under a dollar. Even earning minimum wage, it takes a worker five minutes to earn enough money to buy adequate calories for two full days.

All of this means that Americans are simply eating too much, all the time, every day. They snack too much. They eat meals that are too large, made up of ingredients that are calorie dense, at speeds far too rapid to allow a normal satiation response to be activated. The only solution is to eat smaller portions, eat less frequently, and eat foods that are less fatty, sugary, starchy, and salty.

The food industry and well-meaning (but wrongheaded) poverty advocates have consistently suggested that the answer to these ills is for Americans to eat *more*, but more of foods that are healthier, such as fruits and vegetables. For a generation, the USDA has issued its recommendation to "strive for five" portions of fruits and vegetables each day. First Lady Michelle Obama emphasized similar goals with her organic vegetable garden behind the White House, and a whole vocabulary of food "deserts" has grown up among poverty advocates who postulate that the problem with obesity in poor communities comes from a lack of access to fresh fruits and vegetables.

But research does not bear any of this out. There is little evidence that Americans are suffering ills from eating too few vegetables. The Inuit, for example, eat virtually no vegetables and have relatively low rates of heart and vascular disease or colon cancer.[32] Various studies of consumer reactions to new, better supermarkets with larger produce selections show that neighborhood residents do not respond by buying and eating more vegetables. (The observed increase is as little as one-quarter of one serving more per day.)[33] One food researcher, Helen Lee, admitted that after multiple such experiments, "What children had access to in their residential environments didn't predict who became overweight or who stayed overweight."[34]

That is, the food desert proponents have their causality wrong. Poor people do not eschew fruits and vegetables because nearby groceries do not stock them. Rather, grocery stores in poor neighborhoods do not stock fruits and vegetables because their customers do not want to buy them. Regardless, the problem is not really one of eating too few vegetables. In theory, more vegetables in the diet could displace more caloric alternatives, but in practice, they do not. People simply eat too much and continue to eat as long as food is placed in front of them. Eating more vegetables does not put a brake on consumption. The more effective response would be to produce, process, serve, and consume less of *everything*. A team of food researchers concluded pithily, "The overconsumption of discretionary calories was much greater than the under consumption of fruit and vegetables."[35]

SNACKING

Ever-present, ultra-palatable food would be less of an issue if we were to cleave to traditional eating rites, but we do not. In the past generation, *snacking* has crept into American lives such that the typical American adult now eats four and a half meals a day, and the typical child eats five.[36] Snacks have gotten bigger and more calorie-dense, with chips and cakes displacing fruit and sandwiches. From 1975 to 1995, calories from snacks grew from 11 percent of daily intake for Americans to nearly 18 percent.[37] This "grazing" approach to life, in which food creeps into progressively more non-meal situations—spectator events, business meetings, athletic practices and games, theater attendance, and driving—adds calories to our diets without inducing compensating calorie reduction at meals. And the trend grows worse.

Many societies recognize that children grow hungry long before the evening meal, and even in France, where snacking is highly frowned on, parents give their child a snack in the mid-afternoon. However, historically, that snack was understood as a crutch for children only and distributed only at a traditional time. "Food is not provided on demand," writes expatriate Karen Le Billon, who is married to a French husband and learning French norms of child-rearing. "Food is provided when adults decide it should be provided."[38] Kessler found the same thing. He discussed the phenomenon with an obesity researcher at Hôtel-Dieu de Paris. "In France, we still have a very strong meal structure," asserted the researcher. "There's a cultural notion that you don't eat between meals?" asked Kessler. "That's right. You don't do that. You learn very early on as children that you just don't do that."[39]

However, in the United States, snacking has grown from a once-per-day ritual for children to a continuous cycle of eating throughout the day for people of all ages. In part, this is due to the breakdown of a traditional meal and household structures as detailed previously, but in part it is also traceable to the omnipresence of food in today's environment. Snack food today is sold nearly everywhere, from gas stations to hardware stores to newspaper kiosks to drug stores. One research team surveyed non-grocery retailers and found that food was sold in 41 percent of *all* retail shops, including furniture and apparel stores.[40] Department stores now sell chocolates next to the underwear racks, and hardware stores sell coffee and donuts at the checkout lines. My local Home Depot now hosts a Dunkin' Donuts inside its front entrance, so that you can now fill up on crullers on your way to the lumber aisle.

Most insidious are the "pouring rights" that soda companies have negotiated with public school systems. While various companies had long negotiated franchise monopolies on college campuses and inside sports venues, primary and secondary schools had been off-limits, due to the perceived harmful effects of soda on kids. However, starting in the late 1990s, school systems leased space in middle and high schools to vending machine operators, bringing soda to students who previously had consumed only water or milk on school grounds. This product placement was part of a broader marketing strategy by the soda companies to make their products ever more ubiquitous; hardly a commercial structure stands in America today that does not harbor at least one soda machine.

Soft-drink marketing strategies have been remarkably successful; our consumption of sugar-sweetened soda increased from twenty-two gallons per person in 1970 to forty-two gallons in 1997.[41] One officer at Pepsi-Cola admitted that selling soda to school kids was a "pretty high stakes business development," and a Coca-Cola representative said of his company's strategy: "We want to put soft drinks within arm's reach of desire."[42] Such ubiquity has its payoffs (for the snack and soda companies) but also its costs. In theory, while any consumer can choose not to consume, in reality people's eating choices are highly influenced by food availability. It takes effort and energy to resist highly palatable and proximate food. When candy and soda machines, and candy counters and donut bars, are present everywhere, the default is to indulge. One cognitive researcher stated the problem thus: "The way society is today, the only way most people can maintain a healthy weight is with active cognitive control—that is, they are thinking about it most of the time."[43] Deborah Cohen agrees: "In my view, the problem is less about access to healthy food than it is about being inundated with too much unhealthy food."[44] As we will see in Chapter

8, this sort of cognitive control requires effort, which tires the cognitive function. Eventually, almost all of us capitulate.

The effect is heightened with food advertising, which fills the airwaves and internet and inundates children's spaces. A disproportionate amount of food advertising is aimed at children and promotes precisely those products that are least nutritious and most calorie-dense: candy, soda, chips, and other snacks. Companies spend close to $10 billion per year advertising food to kids. In one recent year, Kellogg spent $22.2 million just advertising Cheez-It Crackers.[45] Celebrated nutritionist Jean Mayer observed the phenomenon in the early 1970s, noting that the preponderance of all food advertising promoted neither fish, nor meats, nor dairy, nor produce, but rather snacks, candy, soft drinks, and beer. "If you think about it," he wrote, "the bulk of the food advertising is for . . . the least useful things."[46] One cynical marketing consultant, who proffered his services to school systems interested in securing pouring rates, defended his work: "If you have no advertising in schools at all, it doesn't give our young people an accurate picture of our society."[47]

RELEARNING TO EAT

A partial response to the present epidemic must be for Americans to adjust their eating habits. Our palates have grown overly accustomed to bland, over-salted, over-sugared foods. We have come to associate a distended belly with satiation. Moreover, we have become overly reliant on using food for non-nutritive purposes. That is, we eat at all times of the day, not so much out of hunger, but in response to boredom, frustration, sadness, and anxiety. We have habitualized maladaptive eating patterns, and like all bad habits, we will need to unlearn the old ways to acclimate to new ones.

Americans today frequently view eating as a form of self-expression. We aggressively cleave to choice in our diet, demanding autonomy at mealtimes, control over diets, and oversight over food preparation. The 1970s Burger King jingle, "Have it your way," was a direct expression of this ethos. So, too, are announcements on restaurant menus that the kitchens can accommodate any dietary needs and restrictions. As Americans, we expect nothing less.

However, individuality in eating may be part of our problem. In France, which is one of the few countries in the world that is successfully keeping its weight down, eating is seen as a communal event, "the *collective* enjoyment of a set of dishes," in the observation of expat Le Billon (my emphasis).[48] To achieve this critical social milieu, the French school their children in not simply table manners, but also gustatory habits. French children are expected to eat what is placed before them, and what is placed before them is usually the same food that is placed in front of adults. In France, good manners require participating in the meal served by the host . . . and *enjoying* it. The all-important *choice* in American cuisine—the multiple salad dressings, sides, sauces, and preparations which are *de rigueur* at American restaurants—gives way to a coherent meal.

The social quality of eating, so valued by the French, and historically valued by most other people as well (including Americans), is critical in addressing obesity, because social eating is slow eating, and slow eating is healthy eating. The ten to fifteen minute lag between consumption and satiation becomes toxic when food is wolfed down; gastric sensors must be given time to communicate with the brain. Historically, when most foods consumed were raw, tough, fibrous, and bony, the mere act of consumption was slow enough that the lag posed no challenge to satiation. However, in a world of overprocessed food, where thousands of calories can be drunk and eaten during the time it takes for a traffic signal to change, the lag time has become maladaptive. We simply eat too quickly to allow our system to function as designed.

Social eating is a partial remedy since social habits restrict the pace at which people can eat and the quantity that they can help themselves to. Moreover, social conventions impose more moderate pacing on the meal. It is difficult to eat rapaciously if you are making an earnest effort to participate in a conversation. Time studies prove the wisdom of the strategy. While Americans spend less than an hour eating formal meals each day, the French spend over two hours, with sixty-minute lunches and dinners still standard in most of that country.

Moving toward a culture of slower, more communal eating requires deep commitment and profound change. Communal meals require everybody to be present at the same time, meaning that mealtimes have to take precedence over other demands that cloud our schedules. Not only do Americans find it difficult to create time for formal meals, they often take pride in deprioritizing communal eating. Successful people boast about having just enough time to "wolf down a sandwich at work" or "grabbing a slice of pizza in the car" on the way to their meetings. In the world of

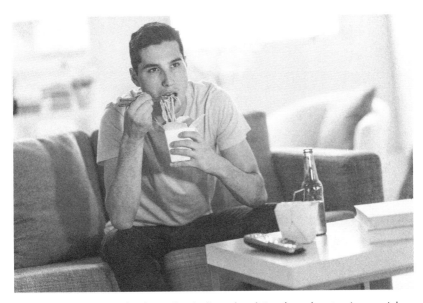

One source of concern has been the decline of traditional meals eaten in a social gathering. Processed food, take-out food, microwavable food, frozen food, and changes in the American family have all contributed to the phenomenon. *Getty Images*

overextended professionals, being called away from the table to take an important call is not so much an inconvenience as a mark of status—the worker is simply too important to devote time to something as frivolous as dinner. However, this delegitimization of meals is wreaking havoc on our waistlines. A partial solution to obesity has to be to elevate eating to an essential daily event, or series of events. Healthy eating is social eating, and social eating requires time and investment.

6

Addicted to Food

FOOD AS A DRUG

For a long time, psychologists and psychiatrists tended to ascribe overeating to psychological causes, such as unresolved anxiety, Oedipal influences, and emotional deprivation. Medical journals in the 1940s and 1950s were filled with references to emotional tension, insecurity, and personality disorders.[1] Hilde Bruch, the nation's foremost obesity researcher in those decades, tended toward Freudian explanations of fat being "protection against men and sex" and food as a stand-in for "love, security, and satisfaction."[2] Physical activity, by contrast, represented "danger, threat, and insecurity."[3]

In a Freudian world, overeating was a learned response to emotional conflict, and as such could be unlearned through psychotherapy and self-awareness. Some psychiatrists spoke of the "fat personality," which could be blunted through psychodynamic catharsis.[4] Benjamin Kotkov, a Boston-based psychologist, used Rorschach inkblots to tease out underlying personality patterns in obese women. Among the common attributes he found in these women were a tendency to daydream, disengage from relationships, and eschew risk-taking. He found in almost all obese women indications of "neurotic personality patterns," which, again, could only be improved through deep therapy.[5]

The problem was mother, of course. Obesity researchers were convinced that most obese adults had grown up in families with overly dominant mothers and distant fathers, and as such, they had failed to adequately separate themselves during adolescence. Frustrated as adults, they turned to food for solace. Perennially unfulfilled, their behavior became self-reinforcing as they further alienated potential friends and mates. In truth, these people needed to "see a psychiatrist before a nutritionist," in the words of Cornell nutritionist Charlotte Young. The right approach, thus, was sympathy rather than scolding. "He is simply satisfying his disordered appetite," explained the leading nutritionist Jean Mayer in 1955.[6]

The problem with these explanations was not so much that they were wrong as that they were unhelpful. Causality was difficult to establish. Many obese people were socially reclusive and insecure, but it was unclear whether the insecurity had caused the obesity, or vice versa. Moreover, while many fat adults had started out as fat children, the cause was again in question. Was the childhood obesity caused by growing up in an emotionally unsupportive household, or had the childhood obesity been caused by a more physiological maladaptation that was continuing to work its ills on the obese adult? Even if there was truth in the idea of overeating as a response to an emotionally stunted childhood, what was to be done? Psychodynamic psychotherapy, the type of therapy that tended to focus on childhood traumas and deep exploration of the psyche, proved nearly useless in correcting poor eating habits. Upon being psychoanalyzed, obese patients may well have gained insight and self-knowledge into their eating, but they tended to stay obese.

Over the next forty years, support for psychological explanations of obesity waxed and waned but never ended. Overeating was non-nutritive eating and thus irrational. In general, when mental health researchers and clinicians saw irrational behavior, they tended to ascribe it to unresolved neuroses or unexamined motives. People were eating for some compelling but non-obvious reason and damaging their bodies, social lives, and careers in the process. The easiest explanation was emotional; people were overeating to satiate emotional needs that in healthy people were met through intimacy, professional and social success, and leisure activities. What other explanation could there be?

However, a small minority of researchers thought that they saw evidence of different motives. Starting in 1950, these researchers noted that the relationship that obese people had with food was quite similar to that which alcoholics had with alcohol: more of a *need* than a desire. Many people enjoyed drinking, but alcoholics seemed to lack control over their drinking. They did not merely *want* to drink; they *had* to drink. Treating alcoholics, as veterans of Alcoholics Anonymous knew well, was far more complex than simply girding them to resist their worse impulses. The treatment had to fundamentally alter their life patterns, changing their friends, workspaces, and even family members to embrace a wholly non-drinking environment. Researchers realized that eating, like drinking, was actually providing "relief" for the obese; it took them "out of the world as it actually was, away from realism."[7]

By 1973, psychiatrist Daniel Cappon was describing overeating as a form of "substance abuse," a new, more inclusive term for drug addiction.[8] Substance abuse included opiates and cocaine but also mild stimulants such as marijuana, prescription barbiturates and amphetamines, and alcohol. And perhaps, according to Cappon, food. Substance abuse was the use of substances to elicit euphoric feelings, or to dull dysphoric ones. Many substances that were abused could be used in a healthy way—using a barbiturate to calm one's nerves before a big speech, for example—but became abused when the user turned to the substance to avoid life's pedestrian challenges or to dull ordinary pain and disappointment. The abuse became addiction when the user lost the ability to live without the chemical crutch.

Cappon and colleagues realized that many obese people were using food in the way that alcoholics used alcohol or that drug addicts used narcotics. They had lost control over their eating and turned to food constantly to cope with ordinary challenges and hurdles. As was true with almost all abused substances, the difference was one of degree. A social smoker could enjoy a cigarette or two at a party without becoming addicted, and most drinkers could do the same with drinking. Many people could enjoy eating rich, satisfying foods without turning to those foods as an emotional emollient or a habitual coping device. The line between ordinary enjoyment and compulsive abuse was hazy but there.

By the turn of the twenty-first century, with obesity rates exploding and no promising therapy in sight, many obesity researchers realized that older explanations relying on psychology or character pathology were simply not useful. However, the idea of overeating-as-addiction was. People who were addicted to food ate all of the time. They ate to celebrate, to drown sorrows, to distract themselves, or to counter boredom. Although almost all wanted to stop, they could not. Some overeaters referred to sugar and carbohydrates as their "drugs of choice."[9] People who were vulnerable to highly hedonistic foods—premium ice cream, pepperoni pizza, french fries—were insatiable; the more they ate, the more they craved. Animal studies reinforced the perception; rats that were denied high doses of sugar after becoming habituated to it actually demonstrated withdrawal symptoms such as anxiety and tremors. David Kessler, the former FDA commissioner, interviewed obese people in front of a table of peanut butter M&Ms, Snickers candy bars, and Little Debbie's snack cakes. One subject, highly distracted by the array, described her feelings: "I do not want them, but I cannot control my desire to eat them. I'm obsessing. I feel totally out of control."[10] Another subject admitted: "I feel very wanton, as if I don't have control over myself, my impulses."[11] Kessler described many overeaters, including himself, as simply "powerless in the face of certain foods."[12]

In the early 1970s, Judith Rodin, a psychologist at Yale, speculated that overeaters responded more intensely to food. Everybody liked to eat, but overeaters *really* liked to eat. She noted that overweight people were sometimes "uncontrollably responsive" to food stimuli.[13] Their pleasure sensors seemed to be more delicately primed, ready to fire explosively at a hint of gustatory reward. At about the same time, Patrick Linton, a psychiatrist at the University of Alabama, noted that normal-weight people lost interest in food after eating, but overweight people continued to be interested. Their pleasure response to eating seemed to be divorced from any objective measure of satiation. Natural overeaters were rarely truly full. The next bite of food continued to tantalize, regardless of how much they had already eaten.[14] Demonstrating this, Stanley Schachter of Columbia University offered subjects crackers after having fed them sandwiches. Normal weight subjects refused the crackers if they had already eaten, but overweight ones did not. They seemed inured to their own level of hunger and satiation, and they continued to find the crackers alluring even if they were not actually hungry.[15]

Recent research on dopamine levels and receptors in the brain suggests that many overeaters have similar brain chemistry to people susceptible to other addictions. These people require a bigger "hit" to their system to produce adequate dopamine to feel good. Normal life experiences are simply inadequate to do this, and thus they turn to chemicals to artificially stimulate dopamine production. Mark Gold, a psychiatrist at the University of Florida, turned to obesity research from tobacco research when he realized that patterns of abuse were quite similar for both food and cigarettes, and he found that smokers who wished to stop smoking frequently found that they had to eat more to maintain a similar psychological equilibrium.[16] Other researchers working with brain scans found identical distortions in dopamine receptors in overweight people. Somehow, overeaters were not experiencing pleasure from everyday experiences in the same way that their thinner peers were.[17]

Of particular interest to many obesity researchers was the relationship of overeating and stress. Stress, the great bugaboo of contemporary life, is toxic. Highly stressed people are far more likely to suffer from heart disease, stroke, and chronic inflammation. They sleep less and eat more. They are less effective at work. They die younger.

People experiencing stress frequently overeat. Researchers theorize that this is not merely a psychological response but rather a neurochemical one. Food, particularly carbohydrates, appears to have a calming effect on many people. Recent research suggests that consuming carbohydrates floods the brain with another neurotransmitter, serotonin, which works to counter anxiety and depression. Judith and Richard Wurtman of MIT have concluded that some people are "carbohydrate cravers," using carbs as a type of antidepressant.[18] One study showed that women eat 20 to 25 percent more calories per day before the onset of menstruation: an unconscious effort to counter the effect of premenstrual depression. Research with rats has demonstrated that animals that are artificially stressed in a lab (through intentional tail-pinching) rapidly grow obese. Their rate of caloric consumption closely dovetailed telltale signs of stress, such as face-washing and nail-pulling.[19] And many studies have demonstrated a consistent gain of eight to ten pounds in people who quit smoking in the first year.[20] In the past, researchers have viewed the overeating after smoking cessation as a quest for oral gratification, but a more recent interpretation is that smokers are simply switching psychoactive drugs: from nicotine to sugar.

Sugar, in fact, appears, to be the key. Sugar, in all of its forms, seems to be particularly psychoactive. Increasingly, it appears to be mildly addictive. While most people through much of history have eaten nearly no sugar beyond what naturally occurs in fruit, people in our time have shown a remarkable ability to quickly habituate to eating enormous amounts of sugar—some 130 pounds per person per year—and growing psychologically and physically dependent on it. Parents and teachers of young children have long observed their charges "crashing" quite rapidly, only to be "picked up" with a quick dose of starch and sugar, but adults appear equally susceptible to the phenomenon.[21] In a further section, we will explore the growing body of evidence of the central role of sugar in obesity, paying close attention to the complex ways that the body metabolizes and stores sugar and signals to the brain to eat more or less of the stuff.

COMPLEX FEEDBACK MECHANISMS

To fully understand the addictive nature of food, it is necessary to examine in some detail the complex ways that the brain, the site of all addictions, interacts with the digestive and fat storage systems to produce feelings of hunger or satiation. It is not at all obvious how these mechanisms work. We are all familiar with the sense of being hungry, and most of us are also familiar with the sense of being sated or full. We eat regularly without being prompted and stop eating long before the food has run out in the larder. Something in our body is telling us through powerful messages to eat and to stop eating.

We tend to think of this feedback process as mechanical. The stomach is a bag that we fill with food several times a day, and it empties itself of that food over the succeeding several hours. When the bag is empty, we feel hungry and eat. When it is full—stretched, bursting—we stop. Moreover, we feel hungry when we lack ready energy (glucose) in our cells, and we eat to replenish our energy reserves.

In fact, the process is substantially more complex. Our stomachs are largely empty most of the time, yet we don't walk around hungry most of the time. At the same time, many of us experience hunger not so much as a physical absence in our gut, but rather as a psychological state of crabbiness, antsiness, and an inability to focus. We often speak of "low blood sugar" or needing a "pick-me-up," and eating does just that. Yet, we often feel substantially better shortly after eating, even when very little of the energy in the food has actually been absorbed into our blood through the small intestine. Something more subtle is governing our hunger and satiation responses.

That something is a series of sensitively balanced hormones that are released and suppressed in response to fat tissue, stomach contents, and energy use. The hormones work in pairs but also agonistically, canceling each other's effects. The system is complicated and gets more complicated as we learn more. Recent research has demonstrated that at least nine hormones and messenger proteins are involved with hunger and satiation, though I will discuss only the most important ones here.[22]

In general, satiation and hunger hormones work on the hypothalamus, an important gland at the base of the brain that is intimately tied to the stomach and gut through the vagus nerve. Hunger and satiation start in the brain, but we *feel* hunger in our gut because of the vagus nerve. We have known that the hypothalamus has a role in hunger since the 1940s when two researchers found that when they destroyed parts of hypothalamus glands in rats, the rats became ravenously hungry.[23] Ten years later, another pair of researchers found that if they removed a different part of the hypothalamus, rats lost their appetites entirely. The hypothalamus has many tasks, but for our purposes here, we can think of it as our master hunger switch.

The most important hunger/satiation hormone to act on the hypothalamus is *leptin*, discovered in 1994 by Jeffrey Friedman and colleagues at Rockefeller University. Leptin is the main satiation signal molecule. It is a protein that is synthesized in fat cells, and therefore its concentration in the blood is correlated not with food intake but with the amount of fat we have. Fatter people produce more leptin and thus, in theory, should be less hungry. Researchers who inject rats with synthesized leptin find that they lose weight rapidly. (Unfortunately, we have not yet been able to safely produce a similar, long-acting effect in humans.) It is important to note that leptin levels do not rapidly change with meals, so leptin's action does not account for our rapid satiation while eating.

Leptin works as a satiation messenger in conjunction with *insulin*. Insulin is a critical metabolic hormone in the body that is produced by the pancreas. Protein receptors on the surface of skeletal muscle, fat cells, and liver cells respond to insulin by allowing glucose to enter those cells. Without insulin, the cells will not receive glucose, and the glucose will remain in the blood to be excreted in the urine. People who don't produce insulin (type I diabetes) or whose bodies are insensitive to insulin (type II diabetes) are enervated because they cannot get glucose into their muscles. Over time, an elevated level of blood glucose in diabetics causes substantial damage to capillaries throughout the body, leading to blindness and peripheral tissue death.

For the purposes of understanding satiation, however, we are interested in insulin not so much for its role in glucose transport, but rather because it behaves similarly to leptin as a satiation signal in the hypothalamus. For many years, researchers did not believe this to be true, since nerve cells (including those in the brain) do not need insulin to be able to absorb glucose. Given that the brain is insensitive to insulin, it seemed counterintuitive to suppose that insulin could work as a satiation messenger on a gland in the brain, but in fact, it does.[24]

Insulin is produced, in part, proportionally to adiposity (that is, the fatter you are, the more insulin you produce), but insulin, unlike leptin, is also produced and released rapidly in response to glucose in the blood. As soon as you eat carbohydrates or sugar, the pancreas releases insulin to transport glucose into muscle cells or, if there is extra glucose, to transport it into fat cells where it is converted to triglycerides (fat). In a secondary reaction, insulin suppresses glucose production by the liver, which is capable of both turning glucose into glycogen and glycogen back into glucose in response to the concentration of glucose in the blood. That is, insulin shuts down the glucose-producing process in the liver while pushing available glucose into muscle and fat cells. And, of course, some of the glucose goes right to the brain without the aid of insulin.

Both leptin and insulin act on a secondary messenger molecule called *cholecystokinin* (CCK) that, in turn, signals the hypothalamus to inform the gut that you are sated. There are other secondary and even tertiary messenger molecules involved as well, but for our purposes, we can focus on insulin and leptin. One more important point that has recently come to light is that large amounts of insulin can actually *suppress* the action of leptin, which may be why we are seeing so much obesity in type II diabetics, who actually produce huge amounts of insulin to overcome the body's growing insulin insensitivity. That is, very fat people are producing large amounts of insulin that ought to act as an appetite suppressant. However, the large amount of insulin is blocking the action of leptin (the primary appetite suppressor), and thus people feel hungry despite having an abundance of stored energy. Even sadder is that all of this excess energy does not make people feel particularly energized, since little of the available glucose can get into the skeletal muscles where it can be burned. Thus, we see a toxic combination of being overweight while feeling simultaneously hungry and exhausted.[25]

Two hormones work agonistically with leptin and insulin to produce feelings of hunger. *Neuropeptide Y* (NPY) is a messenger molecule produced in the hypothalamus that stimulates eating and fat storage while lowering metabolism. It is the starvation molecule, evolved over millennia to keep us focused on finding and consuming food during times of scarcity while lowering our inner burn rate to conserve what glucose we have. People who lose weight have elevated levels of NPY, suggesting that the body detects the lost fat and is signaling the gut to try to replenish it by eating more. NPY's effect on metabolism is one of the factors making it hard for dieters to keep their pounds off; the more you lose, the less you must eat to maintain the same weight.

Most recently discovered, but garnering a good deal of press, is *ghrelin*, the master hunger molecule, discovered by two Japanese researchers in 2000.[26] Ghrelin is produced by the stomach and acts on the hypothalamus.

Ghrelin also causes the stomach to contract, leading to that growling, tight feeling in our gut that we associate with hunger. We are still learning about ghrelin, but its production by the stomach may be the reason why we tend to feel hungry on a regular mealtime basis, even though the time between meals is not long enough for our fat reserves to fall. Subjects who are injected with ghrelin experience extreme hunger urges—one researcher called its effect "amazingly powerful."[27] A condition where people produce too much ghrelin, Prader-Willi syndrome (PWS), produces such extreme obesity that sufferers often die before the age of thirty.

Ghrelin may explain the striking success of bariatric bypass surgery, which I will discuss at greater length in Chapter 8. The surgery, in which as much as two-thirds of the patient's stomach is removed, results in rapid weight loss with very little sense of hunger. Frequently (though not always) the weight loss is permanent. Researchers have puzzled over why the surgery has been so successful, given the ability of at least some patients to override the mechanical constraint of having a smaller stomach by constantly sipping high-calorie milkshakes. However, if removing a large part of the stomach also substantially reduces the ability of the stomach to produce ghrelin, the sharp curtailment of hunger might follow.

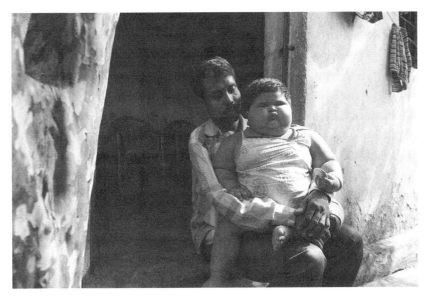

A child suffering from Prader-Willi syndrome, in which the body overproduces ghrelin. Victims are insatiably hungry. Many die very young. *Getty Images*

We are still learning about these feedback paths, and there are probably more intermediary molecules of which we are unaware. Still a mystery is an alternate metabolic pathway we see during times of starvation, in which glucagon, epinephrine, and cortisol work together to produce ketogenesis in the absence of insulin. This might explain why people on long fasts find that hunger pangs vanish almost entirely after the first twenty-four hours. It also might explain why many people find it easier to stick with diets that are extremely low in carbohydrates, such as the Atkins or South Beach diets.

One last point. All of these feedback mechanisms have spurred some obesity researchers to question the basic causal component of obesity: overeating. We know that people who eat too much are often fat, but is it the overeating that is causing obesity, or the obesity that is causing over-eating? In the past, we have assumed that it is the first, but recent insights into hunger and satiation mechanisms suggest that perhaps it is the second. Excess fat produces insulin insensitivity in muscle cells, which causes a glucose deficit in the muscles. The pancreas responds to the shortage by producing more insulin, which in turn blocks the satiating action of the leptin that all of the fat is producing. The hypothalamus, starved of leptin, urges the individual to eat more, even as she finds herself unable to engage in physical activity due to the glucose deficit in her muscles. All of the carefully calibrated feedback mechanisms are being thrown out of kilter for a complex set of reasons.

TOXIC SUGAR

Our feedback mechanisms are out of whack for a variety of reasons, but the rise in our consumption of sugar weighs heavily (pun intended). Ubiquitous sugar, which we now consume at the rate of nearly three pounds per week, came late to our diet. While we have always had a taste for the sweet, for 99.9 percent of our time on Earth, our only source of it was whole fruit, where it was combined with plenty of water and fiber and available only in season. Several hundred years ago, we learned to dry it and concentrate it in the form of preserves and jams, but even these were only half sugar at most and were relatively rare and expensive. Very wealthy people could use bee honey or maple syrup as a sweetener in cooking, but these were prohibitively costly luxuries to be used sparingly, if at all.

Sugar, by which most of us mean granulated sucrose, is a disaccharide ("two-sugar") with one molecule of glucose and one molecule of fructose bound to each other. (In the body, these are cleaved quickly.) Glucose, a simple sugar, is the basic fuel behind all of our metabolic processes. Curiously, it is not particularly sweet when eaten by itself. Fructose, by contrast, is very sweet. It is the stuff that makes fruit and fruit juice sweet. In the body, it is converted to glucose which then enters the muscles and fat cells. Our table sugar is exactly 50 percent fructose and 50 percent glucose. *High-fructose corn syrup* (HFCS) is nearly identical to table sugar, albeit with a touch more fructose (about 54 percent). Honey, cane sugar, raw sugar, and brown sugar are all nearly identical to table sugar, with a few impurities that make them taste slightly different. Powdered sugar is simply finely ground table sugar with cornstarch added so that it sprinkles nicely on cookies. From our standpoint, trying to understand the role of sugar in obesity, hunger, and satiation, all of these sugars are identical. People who use honey to sweeten their tea thinking that they are drinking healthier are deceiving themselves. If it's sweet and it's not artificial then it's sugar.

Nearly all of the sugar that we eat today comes from two plants: sugar cane and sugar beets. While we have known of both for centuries, processing developments in the eighteenth and nineteenth centuries allowed us to extract the sugar from these plants, boil it, purify it, package it, and ship it. Sugar rollers allowed us to squeeze the sugary juice from the highly

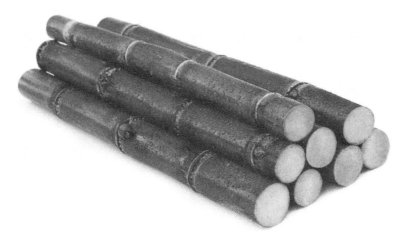

Freshly cut sugar cane. Trying to get the sugar out of it without commercial sugar rollers is akin to chewing on raw bamboo. *Dreamstime Images*

fibrous sugar cane plant in the eighteenth century, and colonization of the Caribbean (the "sugar isles"), coupled with slave labor allowed middle-class Europeans to use sugar regularly starting at the beginning of the nineteenth century. By 1750, Great Britain had 120 sugar refineries consuming the cane output of Jamaica, Barbados, St. Kitts, and the Leeward Isles. Before the American Revolution, tiny Barbados, an island only fifteen by twenty miles in dimension, produced as much wealth as all of Britain's North American colonies combined. At about the same time, German agronomists realized that similar techniques could be used on sugar beets, allowing northern Europeans to produce their own sugar.

Several further accelerants to our sugar consumption came in the form of widely available teas and coffees for the middle class in the nineteenth century (which tasted substantially better with sugar) and also the development by Thomas Welch in 1869 of a process to pasteurize grape juice, thus allowing for its storage and shipment without fermenting it into wine. Grape juice became popular at the turn of the twentieth century, with Prohibition in the United States making it even more appealing. Orange juice

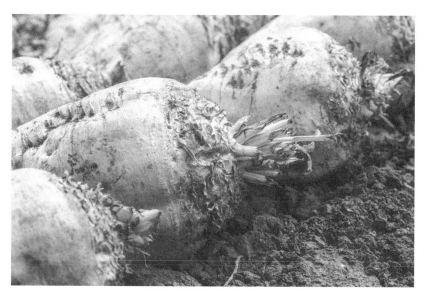

Cultivation of sugar beets in France and Germany in the late eighteenth century allowed those countries to produce table sugar domestically. Use of sugar as an ingredient in cooking, almost unknown before 1750, rapidly rose. Today, we eat a hundred pounds of sugar per year per person and an additional thirty pounds of corn syrup. *Getty Images*

made its appearance after World War II with the same nutritional problems as cane sugar—processing had separated the sugar from the fiber, allowing Americans to hyper-charge their consumption of the stuff. To get as much sugar from unjuiced apples or oranges as from a large glass of juice, you would have to eat five oranges or eight apples in rapid succession. Americans today drink over twenty gallons of orange juice yearly, along with another twenty gallons of apple, grape, and tomato juice. When we add in sugared soft drinks, Americans are drinking nearly 40 percent of all of their sugar.

A further development came with the development and commercial use of high-fructose corn syrup in 1970, which rapidly took its place in soft drinks (10 percent HFCS), salad dressing (as much as 30 percent), tomato sauce (10 percent), ketchup (30 percent), chicken nuggets (6 percent), coffee creamer (60 percent!), and flavored yogurts (40 percent).[28] While our consumption of table sugar has stayed fairly constant for the past half-century at roughly 100 pounds per person per year, we have added an additional thirty pounds of corn syrup to our diets, explaining at least part of the obesity explosion we have witnessed in that time. Today, we can find sugar or corn syrup in a startling array of processed and pre-prepared foods, from hot dogs to crackers, pizza, granola, and Worcestershire sauce. In fact, it is the rare packaged food that is made without sugar. And more packaged foods are getting sweetened all of the time. I was disheartened to find recently that my favorite brand of frozen fish fillet is now being breaded in sugared breadcrumbs.

Although a growing number of nutritionists and endocrinologists believe that sugar is the most significant dietary factor in the rising obesity rate, this consensus has come very recently and is still not complete. In fact, for much of the last half-century, most dieticians and nutritionists believed that dietary fat was the principal culprit in obesity and heart disease. The individual most responsible for this conjecture, physiologist Ancel Keys, spent much of his career attempting to prove just this. Keys noticed in the 1950s that rates of heart disease were substantially lower in the war-torn nations of Europe than in the United States, and he hypothesized that the cause was reduced consumption of animal products—particularly fats. He paid specific attention to the unusually long-lived residents of southern Italy and, noticing that their diet contained few animal fats, looked elsewhere for confirmation. His widely read research on heart disease in seven countries (the *Seven Countries Study*) began in 1958 and demonstrated a correlation between consumption of animal products and rates of heart disease in Japan, Italy, England, Wales, Australia, Canada, and the United States. Keys spent the rest of his career advocating strongly and effectively for reduced consumption of red meat and fat.

Keys's recommendations were fueled by the publication in 1977 of *Dietary Goals of the United States*, a major report on nutrition and health produced by the Senate Select Committee on Nutrition and Human Needs (often called "The McGovern Committee," after its chairman). *Dietary Goals* recommended, a la Keys, that to reduce the chance of heart disease and obesity, Americans should eat fewer eggs and less dairy and meat while consuming more complex carbohydrates. The publication of the report sparked a mass anti-fat movement in the United States, impelling food producers to create many new low-fat products, often with greater amounts of sugar added to make up for the flavor lost in the fat. Americans successfully cut their fat intake but at the cost of eating more sugar. Obesity rates rose concomitantly.

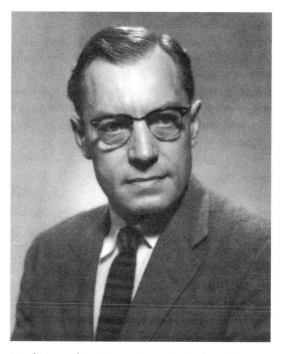

Ancel Keys, whose *Seven Countries Study*, published in 1958, promoted the notion that dietary fat was the main culprit in heart disease and obesity. *University of Minnesota Archives*

Robert Lustig, an endocrinologist at the University of California in San Francisco, has devoted substantial time and effort in debunking Keys's findings. Lustig is particularly critical of the fact that Keys selectively chose seven countries that validated his findings while ignoring heart disease rates in an additional fifteen countries that did not. Furthermore, Lustig believes that Keys was inadvertently selecting for countries that were consuming large amounts of *trans* fats (mostly in the form of Crisco, margarine, and other artificially hydrogenated vegetable oils), which *are* implicated in heart disease. It was an unfortunate happenstance that in the late 1950s, when Keys was conducting his research, many wealthier countries that were consuming large amounts of animal products were also consuming large amounts of trans fats.[29]

However, even in the midst of the low-fat craze, many lesser-known nutrition researchers produced findings at odds with Keys's hypothesis. In 1951, for example, Otto Schaefer, a physician from Germany, studied Inuit natives living on Baffin Island in far Northern Canada. The Inuit traditionally lived on a diet composed entirely of meat and fish, but by the early 1950s, a few communities were supplementing their diets with imported processed foods that were high in sugar and carbohydrates, providing perfect research conditions. Schaefer found that the Inuit who maintained their traditional diet were nearly totally free of heart disease, atherosclerosis, and gut ailments, while those who supplemented their diets with carbohydrates suffered from tooth decay, diabetes, rising obesity, and high blood pressure. Schaeffer described the Inuit's move to a Western, sugar-laden diet as "self-inflicted genocide."[30]

Other researchers observed similar changes in health when people who had previously cleaved to traditional foods adopted Western-style, sugar-laden diets. One team of researchers removed a group of diabetic Australian aborigines with risk factors for heart disease living outside of Derby to their tribal lands where they were denied access to all Western foods. There, they transitioned to a traditional diet based almost exclusively on seafood, bush meat, grubs, and tubers. In only seven weeks, members of the group lost an average of eighteen pounds and displayed significantly lower blood pressure.[31] In another study in the early 1970s, researchers in Israel observed the near total absence of diabetes, high blood pressure, and heart disease among recent Jewish immigrants from *mizrachi* (North African and Middle-Eastern) communities, which stood in marked contrast to relatively high rates of heart disease and obesity in immigrant Jews from *ashkenazi* (Central and Eastern European) communities. The mizrachi

Jews consumed carbohydrates but virtually no sugar in their traditional diets. Upon moving to Israel and adopting sugary ashkenazi diets, incidence of heart disease in the community jumped from eighteen deaths per 1,000 to ninety-four deaths per 1,000, virtually identical with rates for the ashkenazi Jews.[32] One of the researchers concluded from the study that calories from sugar should not exceed 5 percent of daily calorie intake, rather than the 50 percent common among Westerners.[33]

Other studies suggested that many different diets—relying, respectively, on fats, dairy products, seafood, rice, whale blubber, salted vegetables, raw cow blood, and pork—could *all* produce salubrious results. Swiss farmers, for example, ate diets heavy with full-fat dairy products and fatty meats, yet they showed little incidence of obesity or heart disease. Researchers observed similarly low levels of heart disease and obesity in Samburu tribesmen of northern Kenya (who subsisted almost entirely on milk and meat); the Masai in Tanzania (similar diets to the Samburu); Eskimos in Greenland (though not Eskimos who had moved to Denmark); and Irish residents of small Irish villages (though not Irish residents of Boston). Diets for all of these relatively healthy people varied greatly, but in every case, they contained little or no sugar.[34] Moreover, in each case where a subset of the native population adopted a Western diet, rates of obesity, heart disease, and atherosclerosis quickly rose.

Mainstream scientists were aware of these phenomena from the late 1950s, yet were reluctant to dismiss the Keys's thesis. As early as 1961, The US Department of Agriculture listed sugar as a risk factor in heart disease and atherosclerosis and recognized the danger of substituting juice and soft drinks for water.[35] In 1962, the report of the Nutrition Education Conference in Washington, DC, recommended cutting sugar and increasing vegetables and whole grains.[36] Moreover, in 1972, John Yudkin, a British physiologist and nutritionist, published his landmark *Pure, White and Deadly*, summarizing his work of twenty years and arguing that sucrose was directly implicated in diabetes, obesity, heart disease, and high blood pressure.[37] Finally, in 1988, chemists at the USDA's Human Nutrition Research Center in Beltsville, Maryland, conducted a controlled experiment in which twenty-one men were fed a diet artificially high in fructose but similar in all other ways to a typical American diet. After five weeks, all of the men showed elevated levels of LDL ("bad") cholesterol, triglycerides, and uric acid—all risk factors for heart disease, atherosclerosis, and diabetes.[38]

Sugar alone does not explain the obesity epidemic, but it is an important component of it. Returning to the theme of this chapter, sugar is dangerous, in part, because of its toxic effects on our homeostatic weight control mechanisms and endocrine system but also in part because we love it so much. Fructose, particularly, seems to do an end-run around our delicately calibrated ghrelin/leptin feedback cycles. When we drink sugar-laden soft drinks, for example, the sudden influx of energy does not seem to disable the ghrelin-producing mechanism as other calorie ingestions do. Our gustatory-pleasure sensors, adapted to lead us to fruit and yams, have been hijacked by the highly concentrated fructose that now suffuses our diet in the form of refined sugar and corn syrup. It is similar to stimulating our natural opiate receptors, designed to detect faint traces of natural opiates in our bodies, with pure heroin. The heroin produces an instant addicting euphoria that our receptors were never intended to handle. Few of us could resist the siren call of near-free, legal, ubiquitous heroin, and even fewer of us can now resist the allure of omnipresent sugar.

Soft Drinks

Readers interested in the dangers of sugar are familiar with nutritionists' diatribes against soft drinks. Soft drinks pose a health threat not because they are uniquely dangerous, but because they are beguiling. Americans now drink over 40 percent of all of the sugar in their diets in the form of either fruit juice or soda, and yet most of those who indulge are ignorant of the volume they are imbibing.

Sugar-sweetened carbonated water was created just over a century ago when an enterprising soda jerk at the Jacobs Pharmacy in Atlanta, Georgia, serendipitously mixed the soda water he was drawing for customers with a locally sourced stomach tonic—Dr. Pemberton's French Wine Coca: a concentrated syrup made of sugar, cola-nut extract, vanilla, and diluted cocaine. The mixture was intoxicating, energizing, and deliciously refreshing in the hot Georgia summers. It became an immediate local hit and inspired other sorts of sweetened soda waters flavored with sassafras root, orange syrup, celery seed, raspberry juice, strawberry juice, grape juice, and pretty much every other fruit flavor people could think of. Invariably, the more sugar that druggists added to the mixture, the more people liked it. It was extraordinarily cheap to make, being largely tap water and sugar, and the proprietary syrups could be transported to distant bottling facilities and mixed with water there. Once regulators removed the cocaine, health officials and doctors gave their blessing, as did ministers, priests, army commanders, and school teachers. Hardly a critic could be found. It remains the favorite indulgence of tobacco-free, alcohol-free Utah. It has become an all-American icon and travels with our troops to all corners of the world.

Children love soda, and harassed and financially strapped parents are happy to oblige them. (Teenagers have lately been turning to "sports drinks"—a category of sugar-sweetened beverages that also include salt and potassium.) A large three-liter bottle of generic soda (which is nearly indistinguishable from the more expensive national brands) can be had for as little as $1.50—about a fifth the price of a comparable amount of milk. And while about a quarter of all soda drunk today is sugar-free, that still leaves about 1.5 pounds of sugar pouring into our stomachs each week.

There is little evidence that drinking sugar is any worse for you than eating sugar, so some of the criticism of sugared drinks is overstated.[39] But we tend to drink sugar faster than we eat it, and liquids appear to by-pass a principal mechanical satiation mechanism of physical fullness; the stomach simply empties itself of fluids too quickly for the engorged feeling to signal us to stop indulging. So drinking sugar really exacerbates the broader problem of eating too many highly processed and hyper-palatable

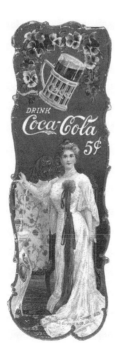

The original Coca-Cola, sold in seven-ounce bottles for a nickel. For thirsty Southerners at the turn of the twentieth century, the soft drink proved wonderfully refreshing. *Getty Images*

calories in which fiber has been removed and thus the pacing of consumption thrown off. It is simply too easy to drink a huge quantity of sugar very quickly, almost without thinking about it.

The commercial food industry understands how inexpensive it is to inflate soft drink sizes (to infinity, really, with the refillable fountain drink sold at many fast-convenient restaurants), and super-sized drinks are now ubiquitous. Nutritionists and public health advocates have taken sharp aim at soft drinks because they appear to be such an easy component of our diets to change. After all, potable tap water is ubiquitous in the United States, and it is essentially free and often tasty. (New York City tap water frequently beats out bottled waters in blind taste tests.) Yet the public has resisted these entreaties. When Michael Bloomberg, mayor of New York City, tried to pass legislation in 2012 limiting soft drink sizes sold at restaurants to sixteen ounces, the proposal was rebuffed as the product of overly intrusive governance. (I discuss this further in Chapter 9.) Americans, it seems, are not yet willing to cede their inalienable right to poison themselves and their children.

Sugar Policy

The sugar industry has held two principal objectives in its dealings with the government for the better part of a century: keeping its price high and deflecting public concerns over its potential insalubrious health effects. The United States grows most of its own sugar in Louisiana, Georgia, and Florida, and supplements its cane supply with sugar from sugar beets. As labor has always been one of the principal costs in producing sugar, poorer countries with cheaper labor (such as Cuba and the Philippines) always threaten to undermine American growers.[40]

The growers' response has been protectionism. In 1934, Congress passed the Sugar Act which placed quotas on sugar from various countries, guaranteeing sugar growers in Louisiana and Hawaii a substantial portion of the US market despite high labor prices. The Act imposed a tariff on sugar importation and kept US sugar prices about 30 percent higher than prices in comparable industrialized countries. Multiple amendments over the following decades showered largesse on Haitian growers (a reward for fealty to the United States) and punished Cuban growers. And the tariffs acted as a substantial subsidy for US growers.[41]

Sugar producers learned through protectionism the power of lobbying. In the early 1960s, Venezuela hired lobbyists to raise its sugar quota in the

United States. In response, the Committee on Agriculture in the US House of Representatives raised the Venezuela quota twelvefold from initial administration recommendations while cutting Argentina's quota by two-thirds. Notably, Argentina had failed to hire a lobbyist.[42]

In the following decades, sugar and processed food producers directed their lobbying dollars in a different direction: toward convincing the American public that sugar was not unhealthy. The sugar industry hired spokesmen in the 1970s to tout its message that sugar was "one of our cheapest sources of food energy," while the cereal manufacturer, Kellogg, claimed that sugar-sweetened cereal was "a solution to some world hunger problems."[43]

Big Sugar (as the industry was often known) worked hard to inject sugar into the US Department of Agriculture's food "pyramid" of recommended foods through the 1980s and 1990s, and in 2004, they lobbied Congress to withhold funding from the World Health Organization after that group recommended that calories from sugar should make up no more than 10 percent of the diet.[44] The USRDA statistics found on all packaged food in the United States does not list the daily recommended amount of sugar that one "portion" of a product provides (in contrast with statistics regarding most vitamins and minerals), and the FDA does not require food processors to aggregate the sugars in their products into one listing, creating the common confusion of having sugar listed in ingredients under multiple and often misleading names.

The industry has also funded substantial amounts of nutrition research that, not surprisingly, tends to conclude that sugar is benign. The Sugar Research Foundation—an industry arm—funded research from the 1940s in schools of nutrition, food science, and home economics to prove that sugar was not only not harmful but, rather, was an important component of a healthy diet. One grantee in 1945, for example, took $7,400 from the industry to study the "protective action of sugar against cirrhosis of the liver."[45]

Perhaps the industry's most insidious effort has been its funding of nutrition research at schools of public health and nutrition. To cite one example, Frederic Stare of the Harvard School of Public Health, perhaps the nation's most well-known nutritionist in the 1960s and 1970s, routinely concluded that sugar was harmless. (He made similar claims for DDT and saccharine.) He also rebuffed calls for Americans to eat more whole grains and to eschew bleached flours and rice. Funding for his lab came from (among others) Beatrice, Campbell's, Coca-Cola, Gerber, Heinz, Nabisco, Nestle, PepsiCo, Stouffer's, and Lipton. In a joint study with the Harvard Dental School, Stare concluded that sugared cereals did not cause tooth decay. The study had been funded by Kellogg.[46] Stare, the son of a Wisconsin cannery owner, trusted large food companies. One reporter mused that Stare was "still a food processor at heart."[47]

Lobbying money has distorted public perceptions of sugar, and it has been responsible for shielding the industry for decades. While other toxic indulgences are closely regulated—tobacco and alcohol among them—sugar continues to be sold free of regulation. Any person of any age can walk into a store at any time and buy as much sugar and sugar-laden products as he or she desires. Proprietors are happy to sell young children large sodas and jumbo packages of candy despite conclusive evidence that youthful indulgence in such treats can lead to a lifetime of habituation, dependence, and multiple chronic health effects. We seem to be recapitulating our war against tobacco of fifty years ago when only an enlightened and scientifically literate few understood the dangers. When it comes to sugar, most of the population has bought the industry line.

Notably, wealthier and more sophisticated consumers *do* sharply limit their own sugar consumption, and they use their wealth and influence to regulate sugar consumption by their kids. Parents in wealthier school districts lobby to get candy and soda machines out of the public schools, keep fast-food restaurants from opening near their homes, and subsidize healthy lunches and snacks for their kids. One of the dominant themes of this book is that the ultimate solution to fighting obesity is changing our environment, and currently, we see the wealthy doing exactly this—creating micro-food environments with reduced amounts of sugars and processed foods in the institutions where they and their children work, play, and learn. However, when Congress has tried to regulate the presence of sugar and processed food in the broader environment, it has been rebuffed. With billions of dollars in sales at stake, and a public not yet willing to recognize the dangers that these foods present to them, the industry is winning the battle over our environment.

DIABETES

Most people today are somewhat aware of sugar's dangers through its association with diabetes. *Diabetes*, from the Latin "to flow through," was named for its most obvious symptom: the unslakable thirst of its sufferers, and their constant need to urinate. Early physicians coupled the copious urination with accompanying wasting away of muscles and bones and suspected that the tissues themselves were being egested with the urine. In the sixth century, physicians recognized that the urine of diabetics tasted sweet; a thousand years later, they concluded that the sweetness was born of glucose in the urine and added a second name to the disease: *mellitus*, from the Latin *miel* (honey).[48]

In 1889, Oscar Minkowski and Joseph von Mering discovered that removing a dog's pancreas caused it to rapidly grow ill. One story goes that a lab assistant observed flies being attracted to the urine of the dog that had undergone the procedure.[49] However, efforts to feed diabetics pancreatic extracts failed to work. (We now know that pancreatic extract, or insulin, is denatured in the stomach and rendered ineffective.) In 1921, Frederick Banting and Charles Best, two researchers working at McGill University, found that injections of pancreatic extract could ease symptoms in diabetic dogs. The discovery quickly led to commercial production of cow insulin by the Eli Lilly and Company, and this allowed human diabetics to live substantially longer lives. Insulin-treated diabetics still went blind and lost nervous sensation in their extremities over time, but the time was much more elongated. We now know that even with regular insulin injections, blood glucose levels in diabetics varies far more than it does in non-diabetics and thus causes slow but irreparable damage to capillaries throughout the body.

Initially, diabetes was mostly observed in patients who lost pancreatic function as children and were wholly unable to produce insulin. We call this disease *type I* or *juvenile onset* diabetes. However, a second class of people developed diabetic symptoms as adults, often in their fifties and sixties, after having lived for decades without it. These patients were almost always obese. The problem for them was not a lack of insulin; in fact, they often produced large amounts of insulin. Rather, as observed by Jesse Roth and Ronald Kahn of the National Institutes of Health in the 1970s, the cells of these patients had grown insensitive to the action of insulin. These patients suffered from *adult onset* or *type II* diabetes, and they frequently were able to ameliorate their symptoms by losing weight, eating less sugar, and taking drugs to stimulate the pancreas. Until recently, type II diabetes has been relatively rare.

In today's obesogenic environment, however, 90 percent of all diabetes is type II. The incidence of type II diabetes has increased in people over the age of forty by 40 percent and in people in their thirties by 70 percent in the last generation. Among Americans of Hispanic and Polynesian descent, incidence runs as high as 20 percent of all adults. In the Pima Indians, it tops 50 percent. It is growing in all groups, most frighteningly among obese teenagers. Type II diabetes is a chronic disease, with many sufferers able to carry on normal lives through diet adjustment and insulin injections. But in the long run, as is true with type I sufferers, type II kills. Type II diabetics are at increased risk for cancer, heart attack, stroke, blindness, neurological disorders, and dementia. Diabetes is correlated with premature cell aging and brain-stem death.

Recent work suggests that sugar, particularly fructose, is heavily implicated in diabetes, even beyond its obesogenic action. Unlike glucose, fructose is not absorbed in muscle cells through an insulin-mediated pathway. Rather, it is absorbed directly into the liver, where it is used to make ATP. When ATP levels are saturated, remaining fructose is converted to fatty acids, leading to fatty liver syndrome. The liver itself becomes insensitive to insulin, leading the pancreas to produce more, creating more fat storage in adipose tissue. That is, fructose ingestion is a causal pathway to obesity.

In a healthy person, insulin binds to receptors on cell membranes, signaling the cell to release transporter proteins that will capture glucose. For many years, researchers thought that obesity interrupted the action of the insulin receptors. We now believe that the reception sites function normally but that the transporter proteins in the cell, particularly adipsin and glut 4, are blocked by certain proteins produced by adipose tissue.[50]

Fructose is particularly obesogenic because by going directly into the liver in an unmediated pathway, it fails to hit any of our satiation or hunger trigger proteins—leptin, ghrelin, or insulin. You can eat and drink fructose all day with no sense of reaching a limit or being full. This is odd when we consider that fructose is a naturally occurring sugar (it is found in all fruit) and that virtually all land animals eat it when they can. Clearly, we have evolved to eat fructose without it killing us.

The explanation to the puzzle lies in the periodicity of fructose in the wild. Fructose is only available when trees are fruiting—usually only a few weeks a year. Within a month, the fruit has been eaten or lies rotting on the ground. However, during that month, many land animals (and all primates) gorge themselves on fruit. When we talk about bears fattening themselves up for the winter, their primary fattening agent is the berries of late summer. Chimpanzees and baboons will seek out fruiting trees and spend hours eating. It appears that in an effort to allow us to gorge ourselves on fruit during the few weeks a year that it is available, we evolved an ingestion circuit that bypasses satiation. When the fructose is available, we are programmed to eat it non-stop, with the expectation of using the stored fat to survive the lean months ahead.

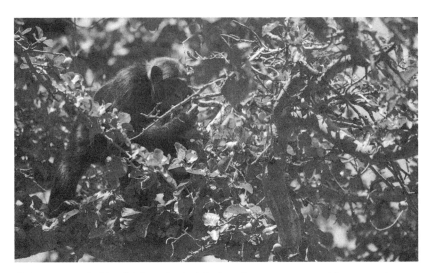

Chimpanzees "fruiting." When the fruit is ripe, the apes can spend hours gorging themselves. Humans have inherited the chimpanzee's ability to bypass the satiation mechanism when eating sugar. *Duncan McKay/Alamy Stock Photo*

In today's sugar-laden environment, however, the fruiting never stops. We are surrounded by cheap fructose every day of the year, and our missing off switches have become a liability. Moreover, few of us can abjure the lure of cheap sugar without expending substantial psychic energy—itself a limited resource. An advantageous loophole in our satiation feedback for most of our evolutionary history has become our undoing. Obesity results, and for many, diabetes follows.

We do we not all get type II diabetes, however. Obesity does not always cause insulin insensitivity in cells. In fact, there is a strong genetic component to type II diabetes; children of two type II diabetics have a 70 percent chance of getting it themselves. To be clear, even individuals with a genetic propensity toward diabetes will rarely get it if they remain thin, but obesity, in combination with susceptible genes, leads inevitably to insulin resistance. Certain groups of people are particularly vulnerable, among them Polynesians, Australian aborigines, Native Americans, and pockets of people in southern India. For some of these groups, diabetes has become epidemic. But type II diabetes is on the rise the everywhere. Researchers estimate that by 2025 the world will have 333 million diabetics and 472 people with pre-diabetic insulin resistance. In 2003, by contrast, there were only 194 million people in the world with either syndrome.

7

Finding the Off Switch

THE FUTILITY OF IT ALL

Who among us does not wish to be thin? That "superb, empty feeling when belt buckle seems to click against the backbone," in the words of a successful dieter in 1953. "Being able to slide both hands inside your waistband. Sliding down from size 18 to 16 to 14 to 12. Friends exclaiming how 'well' you look. They're too jealous to say 'slim.'"[1]

In pursuit of thin, Americans have dieted since colonial days, when Alexander Hamilton's wife warned him to avoid starchy foods lest he get too fat in his long days at Treasury.[2] Americans have shared tips, recipes, slimming advice, and secret weight-loss techniques. Almost as soon as food companies began selling processed food, they also sold processed dietetic food that advertised such attributes as reduced fat, reduced salt, reduced sugar, and reduced calories. In the decade after World War II, about 80 percent of US supermarkets added dietetic departments selling saccharin-sweetened gelatin desserts, low-sugar ketchup, and low-calorie chicken fricassee. Sugar-free soft drinks made their introduction at that time, with Kirsch's Beverages creating a hit product with its No-Cal Ginger Ale. Within a half-decade, sales topped 2.5 million cases per year.[3]

Dieting rarely worked, however. The majority of people who lost weight gained it all back within five years. Albert Stunkard, working in an obesity clinic at the University of Pennsylvania in the early 1960s, found that only 12 percent of his obese patients could lose twenty pounds through dieting and that only 2 percent could keep the weight off for more than two years.[4] One endocrinologist summarized his failures: "The statistics are horrible. It's like treating cancer."[5] A writer reporting on obesity in the early 1960s concluded that reducing was, "a war with the will that is rarely won," while thirty years later, an endocrinologist agreed: "A person who maintains even a small degree of weight loss has done an amazing thing."[6] After years of working, in vain, with dieting patients, one exercise physiologist at Duke University admitted, "I'm almost convinced that dieting is totally useless."[7]

Repeat dieting was even more futile. Dieters who lost and regained weight multiple times discovered that their body responded with less sensitivity to dieting with each successive campaign, creating a notorious "yo-yo" syndrome wherein their bodies went into a permanent starvation mode. In a series of disheartening tests in the early 1980s, researchers found that a group of rats placed on a restricted-calorie diet lost excess weight in twenty-one days and gained it back in forty-six the first time. In follow-up efforts, however, the rats took forty-six days to lose the same amount of weight, and they gained it back in only fourteen while on precisely the same diet.[8]

Reflecting on the futility of it all, William Mueller, a lifelong dieter, appealed to the metaphysical poet John Donne: "The flesh that God hath given us is affliction enough, but the flesh that the devil gives us is affliction upon affliction."[9] The best piece of advice that Mueller found in his quest for slimness was a letter that arrived from his pastor: "Did I understand you to say Saturday afternoon that you are on a diet? Just drop to your knees and ask the Lord to help."[10]

CUTTING FAT

It is hardly a conceptual leap to cut fat out of the diet if one is trying to reduce fat on the body. Fat floating on milk, marbling beef, spread on bread, suffused into cheese . . . how could it help but migrate to our own adipose tissue to enlarge our bellies and inflate our visages? Moreover, from the early 1950s, fat appeared to be actively dangerous. American consumption of fat increased rapidly after World War II such that by 1946 Americans were getting over 40 percent of their daily calories from fat—the highest rate in history. By comparison, Japanese men were only getting about 10 percent of their calories from fat at the same time and Italian men only 20 percent.[11] American waistlines expanded in the 1950s, which seemed proof enough of fat's role in obesity.

More troubling was the concomitant rise in heart disease. Savvy researchers noticed that diseased hearts were often accompanied by clogged coronary arteries (the blood vessels that supply the heart with oxygenated blood) lined with cholesterol—a waxy substance found in animal products that is used by the body for cellular construction. Since eating more animal fat raised cholesterol levels in the blood, it seemed reasonable to suppose that eating less fat would ease cholesterol levels and lead to less cholesterol build-up and fewer heart attacks.

Many American became particularly attuned to the threat of heart disease after President Dwight D. Eisenhower suffered a serious heart attack in 1955 that forced him into weeks of convalescence. Although the stricken patient smiled as he posed for a picture from atop Walter Reed Army Medical Hospital, Americans were hardly reassured. Rather, they took a lesson from the President's new low-fat diet (no more pats of butter on his steak or vegetables), and they chose to lower fat on their own.[12] Newspapers and magazines accelerated the trend with reports of studies showing that coronary patients who refused to change their eating habits died in record numbers, and Ancel Keys, whom we met in Chapter

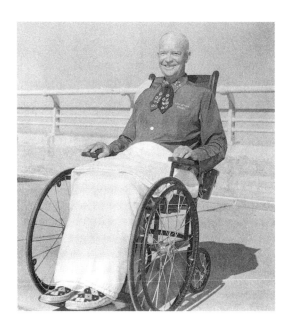

President Eisenhower's heart attack in 1955 focused the attention of many Americans on rising rates of heart disease. Many responded by cutting fat from their diet, as President Eisenhower did while recovering. *Getty Images*

6, trumpeted his own data on the extremely low rate of heart disease in Japanese men who cleaved to traditional diets.[13] Scientists in one study from the mid-1950s extracted lipoproteins from food, centrifuged them to concentrate them, and injected them into rats. Within five hours, the researchers noted accumulation of fatty deposits in the rats' coronary arteries.[14] What could be scarier?

From the late 1950s, concerned Americans began to consciously cut fat from their diet. Grocery stores started stocking "lite" or "low-fat" cheeses and other dairy products, and butchers began to trim their cuts of excess border fat. Ice-cream companies created "ice-milk" products—a sort of milked-up sorbet—while cottage cheese and yogurt manufacturers pushed low-fat and fat-free options. Beef producers who had long prided themselves on producing "well-marbled" (i.e., very fatty) cuts of meat now worked to produce leaner livestock.[15] The movement gained traction with the publication of a major report by the American Medical Association's Council on Foods and Nutrition in 1962 that recommended lowering dietary fat, particularly from animal products. With typical cholesterol for adult American men hovering at 250 milligrams per deciliter (of blood) and heart attacks crippling 1.5 percent of adult American men each year, prudence suggested favoring low-fat products. In New York City, members of the Anti-Coronary Club reduced their dietary fat by 50 percent and recorded a 65 percent reduction in heart attacks over the succeeding decade.[16] Cautious Americans took note.

Although scientists could not produce a precise explanatory mechanism relating fat intake to fat accumulation, the model seemed intuitive. Scientists knew, for example, that fat was the most calorically dense of all foods, so it seemed reasonable that people who ate a lot of fat would gain a lot of fat. Moreover, various studies showed that people who ate a lot of fat seemed to be fatter.[17] The fat-reduction work in the 1960s had produced consistent drops in cholesterol of 10 to 15 percent, and while cholesterol was not exactly fat, it seemed to many people to be a derivative of fat. And, of course, there was the famed Keys seven-countries study which cast a long shadow on dietary fat.

The 1990s produced a cascade of low-fat goods, from Snackwell cookies to special Lean Cuisine prepared dinners to low-fat oleaginous spreads. Even candy companies marketed their wares as low-fat foods, and Americans turned to several low-fat diets, such as one promoted by endocrinologist Dean Ornish that recommended that no more than 20 percent of calories be from fat.[18] One medical advice column suggested ethnic restaurants ("there's always good low-fat food in Chinese restaurants," he wrote[19]) while others pushed rice, sushi, miso, tofu, turkey, and cottage cheese.

The movement's crowning glory was Proctor & Gamble's famed synthetic fat substitute Olestra, invented in 1968 and approved as a food additive by the FDA in 1996. The macro-molecule, in which fatty acids were attached to sucrose to create a molecule too large for normal enzymes to cleave, replicated the mouth-feel of traditional fats while passing undigested through the gut. Proctor & Gamble, along with Nabisco and Frito-Lay, experimented with incorporating the product into a variety of prepared foods, but in the end, they achieved only minimal success. Americans were leery of the "Frankenstein food" created in a lab, and many consumers found that it caused diarrhea.[20] Moreover, the additive appeared to limit people's ability to absorb certain vitamins from food, leading to concerns about malnutrition. Marion Nestle, a nutritionist and staunch opponent of Olestra, noted that consumers did not need new food products "beyond the approximately 240,000 already on the market."[21]

The real problem with low-fat diets was that they did not seem to be particularly effective in helping Americans to get less fat. Through the low-fat craze of the 1990s, when Americans turned to low-fat cookies, ice cream, and TV dinners in record numbers, Americans actually gained weight. From 1980 to 1998, the exact years when Americans were cutting their fat intake most sharply, obesity rates rose from one-fourth of the population to one-third. Low-fat diets were notoriously difficult to adhere to. Nutritionists found that cutting fat to less than one-third of caloric intake was unsustainable for most dieters, and this was far short of the 20 percent of calories advocated by low-fat gurus such as Ornish. One study, in fact, found that people lost weight when they actually raised the content of fat in their diet, and a variety of studies showed that people tended to find diets easier to adhere to when they cut calories by limiting carbohydrates rather than fat.[22] To replicate gustatory satisfaction on the low-fat regimens, Americans turned to sugar for solace, negating any caloric loss from the fat reduction. Bonnie Liebman, a dietitian, summed up the low-fat directive: "For us [nutritionists], that's shorthand for a diet high in fruit, vegetables, and grains," while most people used it as a license to indulge in "fat-free cake, cookies, and ice cream."[23]

The cholesterol question was even more complicated. It was true that people who cut fat from their diet tended to lower their cholesterol levels by 10 to 15 percent, but the drops were not consistent. As far back as 1956, a researcher at the University of Cape Town pointed out that Eskimos (Inuit) who ate a diet that was very high in fat actually had extraordinarily low rates of heart disease and very low levels of cholesterol. Thinking that the Inuit might simply have an odd genetic immunity against heart disease, the researcher fed an Inuit diet of seal and fish oil to the local Bantu population and found that rates of heart disease dropped in them as well. When he experimented with adding sunflower oil to the Bantu's diet, he found that this, too, lowered cholesterol.[24] Realizing fats that lacked a complete complement of hydrogen atoms—unsaturated or polyunsaturated fats—were responsible for lowering cholesterol, the researcher began to recommend that dieters become more discerning in precisely which fats they were cutting out of their diets. Fish and vegetable oils seemed to actually enhance heart health, while beef, pork fats, and vegetable oils that had been artificially hydrogenated appeared to degrade it.[25]

A few years later, researchers led by Edward Ahrens at the Rockefeller Institute noticed an association between blood levels of triglycerides and serum cholesterol levels.[26] However, here again, things got curious. Eating more carbohydrates could actually elevate triglyceride levels while eating certain kinds of fats could actually reduce them. One savvy food writer pointed out that it was possible that triglyceride and phospholipid levels in the blood, and not cholesterol levels, were, in fact, the causative agents for heart attacks and the cholesterol was simply a marker. "If that should be the fact," he wrote, "it could be that using measures to change cholesterol levels is like taking aspirin for a headache due to a brain tumor."[27]

Physicians in the early 1960s noted these associations, but they could not reach consensus on dietary recommendations. Unsaturated fats seemed able to protect some patients against heart disease, but eating too many unsaturated fats could still make you fat, and obesity was correlated with higher rates of heart disease. Moreover, when researchers tried to evaluate the salutary effects of unsaturated fats against the detrimental effects of saturated fats, they found that people needed to eat about twice as many unsaturated calories to reverse the impact of the saturated calories. The better advice seemed to be to tell people not to get fat in the first place by moving more and eating less of everything, and then to eat unsaturated fats in limited amounts while eschewing saturated fat.[28] However, Americans were hardly receptive to such a complicated message in 1962.

LOW CARBOHYDRATES

In direct opposition to those advocating low-fat diets were those promoting low-carbohydrate diets. The idea was somewhat counterintuitive but hardly new. As far back as 1946, one nutrition researcher wrote confidently that getting fat was "generally a reflection of a fondness for carbohydrates, since we can readily transform the latter foodstuff into fat."[29] Early low-carbohydrate advocates, such as H. L. Marriott of Middlesex Hospital (England) promoted "lean meat, poultry, game rabbit, hare, liver, kidney, heart, sweetbread [pancreas] . . . salad, tomatoes, beetroot, watercress, and parsley."[30] He also warned weight-conscious eaters from "bread crumbs, flour, french fries, and canned fruit." Although less orthodox than later carbohydrate alarmists (he allowed for boiled potatoes and fresh fruit), Marriott's inclination to avoid carbohydrates by replacing them with large quantities of lean protein became a guiding mantra for succeeding waves of dietitians over the following fifty years.

Low-carbohydrate diets were supported by empirical evidence fairly early. Research from the early 1940s on rats found increased rates of lipogenesis (fat production) in animals fed high-carbohydrate diets.[31] In 1951, Norman Moore and Charlotte Young of Cornell University observed undergraduate women on a variety of different diets, including a low carbohydrate one designed by Margaret Ohlson of Michigan State College that was similar to the Marriott prescription. Moore and Young found that college women adhering to the Ohlson diet lost 2.2 pounds per week, which was far more than students on low-fat diets. Although the diet upset prevailing shibboleths, with its whole milk and marbled beef regimen, dieters found it far easier to adhere to than previous low-fat and reduced-calorie diets. It literally "sticks to the ribs," explained Moore.[32]

Ohlson's dietary recommendations were followed in the next decade by the best-selling book *Calories Don't Count* by Herman Taller, which advocated eating more polyunsaturated vegetable oils and fewer starches and sweets, including fresh fruit. Although one disappointed dieter noted that the title was misleading ("It turns out that the calories that don't count are such items as safflower seed oils . . . these I have never craved."), many people found the high-fat diet more satiating than low-fat ones, and they were thus easier to adhere to.[33] Taller, in turn, presaged the wildly successful *Dr. Atkins' Diet Revolution* by Robert Atkins, which sold millions of copies through the 1970s. Atkins, who attracted substantial media attention by promoting meals of lobster, steak with butter and béarnaise sauce, full-fat cheeses, and avocado stuffed with shrimp, made claims beyond the thinning properties of his diet; he claimed that his diet cured hypertension and diabetes as well.[34] Moreover, while others accused him of quackery—Nathan Pritkin, a vocal critic, called his diet "a monstrosity . . . a malignancy of nutrition"—Atkins produced thousands of satisfied customers who testified to the success of his approach.[35]

These diets raised the question as to whether eating fats actually helped people to lose weight, or were rather simply more satiating and thus resulted, ultimately, in the dieter eating fewer calories. John Yudkin was not a detractor from the diets, but he did note that the term "high-fat" was misleading; "It should be 'low-carbohydrate' diet," he noted.[36] The real dietetic effect, argued Yudkin, came from simply making it easier for dieters to adhere to a lower calorie diet since people soon grew sick of high-fat foods and actually ate less. His carefully collected statistics bore out his conjecture.[37] Atkins largely agreed with Yudkin, although Atkins tended to articulate the point in more of a salesman's terms. "The advantage of my diet is that it is fun," he pointed out. "My patients can eat meat or any other main course in whatever quantity they wish, and they never go hungry."[38]

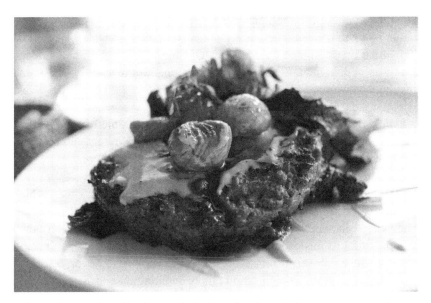

Robert Atkins marketed his low-carbohydrate diet through the 1970s. As seen here, dieters could eat all the protein and fat they wished. Almost everybody lost weight at first, but few could sustain the diet for more than a couple of months. *Getty Images*

The *paleo* diet, which gained popularity in the 1980s, was a further refinement of the low-carbohydrate pattern, albeit one that cleaved philosophically to the diets of neolithic ancestors: high in wild game and fibrous plants with virtually no refined starches or sugar allowed. If Atkins was largely deemed "high-fat" in shorthand, paleo diets were generally referred to as "high-protein." Although the roots of the diet went back to recommendations from the American Medical Association in 1951, it took the odd troika of radiologist S. Boyd Eaton, anthropologist Marjorie Shostak, and internist Melvin Konner to promote the regimen in *The Paleolithic Prescription* published in 1988.[39] The paleo diet drew currency from advances in anthropological research of the time suggesting that earlier humans had eaten radically different diets, which included large quantities of plant fiber (as evidenced by huge jaws), wild game (in days predating domestication of animals), and virtually no starch beyond tubers (as agriculture had only come about 10,000 years before).[40] The idea was hardly crazy, but it ignored the 350 generations of modern humans who had managed to live non-obese lives since the advent of agriculture and animal husbandry. Certainly, the human environment had changed since Paleolithic times, but perhaps the changes germane to obesity were those that had come about in the last fifty years, not the last 10,000.

The Atkins diet worked for many people, at first, but it ultimately proved difficult to adhere to as well. After initially losing weight, many disappointed dieters experienced cravings for starch, and they found themselves nauseous at the idea of eating another meal of cold cuts wrapped around more cold cuts and topped off with a slice of avocado on a slab of brie. The problem was the rigid orthodoxy of Atkins's approach. In the 1980s and 1990s, a number of Atkins knockoff diets were supported by Michael and Mary Eades, Suzanne Somers, and Rachael and Richard Heller, but all promoted diets so low in carbohydrates that many people found them unsustainable over longer periods of time as well. One academic endocrinologist, Xavier Pi-Sunyer, who criticized all of the diets, concluded, "These diets work primarily by making people feel sick."[41]

Ultimately, while many dieters agreed that reducing carbohydrates was an effective part of any successful diet, the nutritional rigidity of most was unsustainable. Research conducted at the University of Pennsylvania in the early 2000s found that after twelve months, weight loss by dieters on an extremely low-carbohydrate diet was not significantly different from that of people on more general calorie-restricted diets.[42] Any diet in which people could reduce their caloric intake over a long period of time would produce reasonable results: The question was what sort of caloric restriction did most people find most tolerable? Endless steak and lobster dinners, fun at first, could prove just as arduous in the long term as ice-milk and low-fat cottage cheese.

STRANGER DIETS

Over the past fifty years, various fad diets have cycled in and out favor, with the banana diet, the buttermilk diet, and the eighteen-day Hollywood diet each having its day.[43] Likewise, desperate dieters sought refuge, at various times in the seawater diet, the fish-and-celery diet, and (a recurring favorite) the yogurt diet.[44] In the annals of kooky dieting, however, none exceeds the ice-cream diet, touted in the late 1960s as the path to "reduce your calorie intake and make pounds disappear." The author of the idea did caution that "regular daily exercise" was probably a good idea to use in conjunction with the diet.[45]

In general, wacky diets restricted the dieter to a particular food group, or even to a specific food, and insofar as they removed appetizing variety from the diet, they worked. That is, most people did lose weight when their food choices were sharply restricted, regardless of what they were limited to. Low-protein diets gained popularity in the early 1970s for this reason, finding form in such odd approaches as the Duke University rice diet in the early 1970s, and other diets where protein was sharply restricted even as sugars and fats were promoted—"patients could have all the butter, sugar, jelly, and rock candy they wanted."[46]

Almost all of these diets worked for a time, but all were unsustainable. Moreover, some of the diets, such as the rice diet, required a residency that *always* worked; virtually anybody could lose weight when they ceded control of their food supply to an outside authority.[47] This was why inmates, prisoners of war, marine recruits, and spa aficionados all reliably lost weight. The challenge was in sustaining the weight loss once the regimentation was removed, and this challenge was actually undermined by the bizarre eating rule that many of these diets subjected their clients to. One thoughtful physician noted in 1956 that for losing weight, "the concept of a single specific factor is not sufficient, since the routine of treatment (limitation in choice of food, fixed times of meals)" was the true proximate cause of the weight loss.[48]

The liquid protein craze of the 1970s took this sort of dieting to a new extreme. Tracing its roots to experimental adult formula supplements popularized in the decade after World War II, millions of Americans starting "drinking" their meals out of a bottle in the mid-1970s, and the vast majority reliably lost weight.[49] Most people who went on liquid proteins consumed 100 percent of their calories in the drink, although some took the protein formula prophylactically before a meal of regular food to dull their appetite.[50]

Liquid protein worked for a variety of reasons. It weaned its adherents from sugar (always helpful) and allowed the diets' designers to adjust caloric intake to very low levels—sometimes as low as 400 calories per day.[51] However, the diet worked primarily because it tightly controlled dieters' food choices. Although this seemed somewhat counterintuitive—the dieter was not being physically restrained, and could easily override the diet by supplementing it with outside food—the severe choice restraint worked. Through the 1980s and 1990s, liquid protein diets retained a small though loyal following, and they inevitably worked provided that the dieters never departed from the diet. Most dieters found that they could not adhere to the regimen, however. They missed the social intercourse that accompanied normal eating and the pleasure provided by food. One professor of medicine summed up the problem with the diets thus: "Behavior modification has to occur in a day-to-day environment. If your only option is to eat the formula, you're not learning about eating cues. It's not like quitting smoking: You don't ever have to smoke again, but you *will* have to eat again. It's not really modification at all."[52]

A variety of diets piggybacked on the liquid protein approach despite being marketed in different ways. The Nutrisystem and Jenny Craig plans both required the dieters to purchase all (or most) of their meals from the company and eat no more than what was provided in the individual portions. Besides the high cost of adhering to these programs, they also failed (as was true with liquid protein) to teach dieters how to cope with a food environment of unlimited choices. Likewise, macrobiotic eaters and health food "addicts" (as they became known in the late 1970s) also sharply curtailed their food choices, often limiting themselves to foods purchased from a particular vendor or from specific farms. These diets were all healthier than the rice diet or the liquid protein diet insofar as they required dieters to purchase and prepare some variety of foods, but all fell short in helping dieters to learn to negotiate the broader food marketplace. The "cancer prevention diet" advocated by Michio Kushi in the late 1980s was described thus:

The diet—a strict macrobiotic approach—breaks down into 50 to 60 percent whole-grain cereals by volume; 5 to 10 percent soup (one to two bowls of soybean-based soup a day); 25 to 30 percent fresh vegetables (but vegetables with tropical or semitropical origins, such as eggplant, potatoes, and tomatoes are excluded unless you live in a corresponding climate); and 5 to 10 percent cooked beans and sea vegetables. All meat is out, only an unspecific "small volume" of fish or seafood a few times a week is allowed, and dairy foods are drastically curtailed or eliminated. Fresh fruit is approved—a few times a week, and only in each fruit's growing season—and dried fruit gets the nod only if it's from the same climatic region as your own.[53]

At least one researcher came to the conclusion that the macrobiotic diet was actually quasi-religious in nature, with its emphasis on *yin* and *yang*, ritualized food preparation, forbidden foods, and metaphysical transformation through eating. Rosabeth Moss Kanter of Brandeis University emphasized the community that formed around the diet and the sacred institutions on which it stood, such as health food stores, certain restaurants and tea shops, and ashrams touting its benefits.[54] The religious component made sense, given the need of these dieters to impose structure on various parts of their lives; Kantor compared some of the macrobiotic followers to Shakers of the nineteenth century and to Hasidic Jews of the twentieth.

However, perhaps the most restrictive (and ultimately the most successful) of these extreme diets was total fasting: no food at all. In 1964, eleven morbidly obese veterans were hospitalized at the Los Angeles Veterans Administration hospital for between twelve and 117 days, and they lost tremendous amounts of weight. One former WAVE (female navy sailor) lost 117 pounds while an army veteran lost ninety-one.[55] Most importantly, after the first day or two, none of the test subjects felt any hunger at all. In the following years, other hospitalized patients were placed on starvation or near-starvation diets, and all lost drastic amounts of weight. In general, men on these regimens lost nearly five pounds per week and women just over three pounds. The attrition rate in most of these programs was low.[56]

Total starvation was obviously unsustainable over the long run, but some physicians and dietitians began recommending intermittent fasting to obese patients starting in the early 2000s. These regimens, which often required patients to adhere to a fast or near fast every other day, also led to dramatic reductions in weight while proving to be more sustainable. Patients on intermittent fasts reported feeling few hunger cravings and did not, as might be expected, overeat on their non-fasting days to compensate for the fast days. Physiologically, the fasts evened out insulin spikes and thus helped wean dieters off of sugar, while psychologically the diets allowed dieters to look forward to indulging on their non-fast days. The approach appeared promising.[57]

Extreme and intermittent fasting both worked to some degree because they removed the element of choice from the dieter's life, and choice in foods has proven highly toxic to many people. This appears to be nonsensical, given the high premium that many of us place on exercising preferences in eating, yet perhaps we ought to pay heed to these successes. Choice in food is a relatively recent phenomenon. Through most of history, we have eaten only foods that were in season, or foods freshly caught, found, hunted, fished, or dug. That is, it is less natural to exercise choice in our eating than we might suppose, and choice (and its accompanying variety) seems to be correlated with obesity. Virtually all of the kooky diets were choice-restricting diets, and most dieters found that they could tolerate the constrained choices while losing weight fairly easily. As we will see in the next section, adding choice back into the diet while maintaining weight loss is the holy grail of dieting, and requires attention, effort, and practice.

SOCIAL NETWORKS

In a sense, the long-term goal of dieting is never to have to diet. That is, rather than put on weight and then have to temporarily put oneself on a weight-reducing regimen, the more sustainable approach is to learn to eat in such a way as to not put on weight in the first place. We all simply have to eat less. I am hardly the first person to propose such an audacious idea. Upon being asked, in 1960, what was the "easiest way for a person to reduce," Henry Sebrell, a widely read physician and dietician, responded merely, "Just eat less of everything."[58] Frederick Stare, his contemporary and colleague, agreed: "It cannot be emphasized too often that the only way to diet successfully is to cut *down* on the total intake of food, not to cut *out* one or two specific foods."[59] And Howard Rusk, the founder of the Rusk Institute of Rehabilitation Medicine, added his own sober note: "No easy way to reduce is safe—no safe way to reduce is easy. The overweight person must learn that only a *permanent* change in his eating habits will bring lasting results."[60]

Permanently limiting portion size is hard, if not impossible, in a food-rich environment. Evolution has tuned appetites and hunger cues to be exquisitely sensitive to available foodstuffs. Most successful reducers find that they have to be constantly vigilant, to the point of near obsession with food. Most ultimately fail. A moment of weakness or shaky resolve can result in hundreds or thousands of extra calories, and for millions of isolated or overworked Americans, these moments come all too frequently.

One promising inspiration to this great challenge has come from Alcoholics Anonymous (AA), the national organization designed to provide peer support and regular social interaction for people trying to resist the call of drink. Alcoholics Anonymous draws on the deep spiritual commitment and resolve of its members but substantially buttresses that resolve with peer pressure. Weekly meetings among AA followers serve to assuage doubts, reinforce good behavior, reward self-abnegation with approval, and provide companionship for those on a long, lonely life quest.

From the early 1950s, a number of dieters and nutritionists noticed that, like alcoholics, people dieting as part of a social group were more successful. In 1950, Edward Rynearson of the Mayo Clinic suggested forming "Calories Anonymous" as a counterpart to Alcoholics Anonymous, while in 1952, researchers observing men on the DuPont Diet noted that much of the success of that diet was owed to the social nature of numerous DuPont executives dieting together. Harold Aaron, a physician and nutritionist, wrote, "Regular meetings of groups of obese persons, under the leadership of someone who has a strong conviction of the desirability of losing weight, can do much to keep up morale required for sustained weight reduction. The element of competitive spirit is also important in this context."[61]

In 1952, the *Journal of the American Medical Association* reported that a group of men who had previously been unsuccessful at losing weight agreed to meet regularly with a leader trained to "stimulate and guide intelligent discussions" about overeating.[62] The group lost substantially more weight when supported by this network approach than it had when each person tried individually. At the same time, a group of women in Milwaukee, under the leadership of Esther Manz, created a "club" to help each other lose weight. Manz drew on her own positive experience in a prenatal class where she observed the women bonding together in a quasi-competitive camaraderie to heed their physicians' prenatal advice. She wondered if the same sort of competitive fellowship could help her and her friends lose weight and, more importantly, maintain the weight loss.

In 1952, Manz founded TOPS (Take Off Pounds Sensibly) as an organization composed of small support groups of dieters. The non-profit achieved substantial success in its early years, and it quickly grew to over a thousand constituent groups waging a "psychological war against acute obesity."[63] TOPS relied on social support and peer pressure and made extensive use of a buddy system where assigned pairs looked after each other and served as a resource for each other in the face of unusual temptation. ("Just about to backslide into a box of chocolates . . ." wrote one amused reporter.)[64] At weekly and bi-weekly meetings, members validated each other's successes, but perhaps equally important, they mocked each other's failings. At several clubs, members who gained weight over a period of time were booed and had to wear a sign cut into the shape of a pig.[65] Oddly, such public shaming did not dissuade people from joining. Rather, it tended to enjoin them to try harder to win the approval of their fellow dieters. If TOPS accomplished nothing else, it proved that social cues were a dominant force in eating behavior.

TOPS was hardly the only peer-dieting group. The California State Department of Public Health experimented with a program of eating support groups at various community hospitals in the 1950s, as did the New England Medical Center.[66] In Denver, the Department of Health and Hospitals began an outreach program to low-income women to both educate them about portion size and food choice and support their efforts at weight loss, with some success.[67] Perhaps most famously, Jean Nidetch, an overweight Brooklyn housewife, founded Weight Watchers in 1963, drawing on a diet

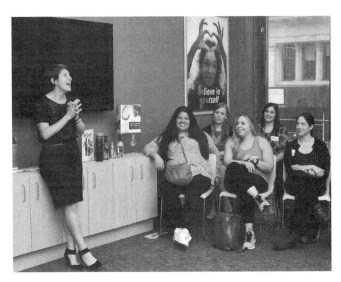

Weight Watchers, founded by Jean Nidetch in 1963, has produced consistent results by inducing people to change their eating habits under the watchful eyes of a group leader and with the encouragement of peers. *Getty Images*

proposed by the New York City Board of Health. In each case, the details of the diet were less important than the social support system of dieters meeting regularly to discuss their challenges and encourage each other to maintain the effort. One dieter admitted after finally maintaining weight loss after a lifetime of failed attempts, "I needed a diet I could follow, and the structure and support of Weight Watchers were important; I couldn't have done it on my own."[68]

Social networks gave millions of dieters the extra support they needed to assert control over their eating. Dieting groups validated the idea that losing weight was *hard*: It was not a task to be taken on lightly, or independently. Relearning to eat at a permanently reduced level was the work of a lifetime that required constant vigilance, encouragement, and even the threat of shaming—thus the weekly public weigh-ins that most dieting clubs subjected their members to. Nidetch, who maintained her 100-pound weight loss until she died, wrote in her memoirs:

> I don't guarantee that losing weight makes life beautiful. I don't guarantee that it's going to give you the success in life that you want. But *surely* it's going to make you confident that you are capable of controlling your own body, that you are not the victim of your compulsions.[69]

TOPS, Weight Watchers, and other groups differed from contemporary kooky and extreme diets because they offered no quick solutions. Rather, they took as their starting point the fact most people needed to relearn lifelong eating habits, identify trigger situations in which they might be tempted to overeat, and learn coping mechanisms to thwart temptation. These groups offered a difficult but sustainable model of dieting. In fact, they did not offer diets at all but rather education and support to help people live the remainder of their lives on reduced portions of everything. That they admitted that losing weight and maintaining weight loss was hard was their first great contribution, and that they persuaded people that few could go at it alone was their second. Thomas Coates and Carl Thoresen concluded, after substantial study, that the best results were achieved with a "high degree of structure and supervision" and included "intensive and frequent individual counseling." They wrote: "It seems very unreasonable to expect to change a long lasting and complex pattern of behavior . . . without intense and sustained time and effort."[70] Healthy weight loss was the work of a lifetime, and it was a team sport. Only the foolish attempted to go at it alone.

8

Exercise, Drugs, and Surgery

EXERCISE

The other side of reducing is burning more calories. Through most of our history, the notion of purposely raising our level of physical activity has been laughable; the energy demands of hunting, gathering, and agricultural work were more than enough to burn everything that could be consumed, and then some. Farmers, loggers, ranchers, and boatmen all reliably burned 5,000 to 6,000 calories daily, and their wives burned only nominally less with their multiple-mile walks to the well, to town, and to the outer pastures, not to mention the physical demands of churning butter, weaving cloth, weeding vegetable rows, and preserving fruit.

However, as we have seen in earlier chapters, the caloric demands of a changing environment and changing labor vastly reduced our need for calories. Office work requires of the average adult male no more than 1,800 calories daily and of the average adult female even less. Unless we artificially raise our caloric needs, we condemn ourselves to a steady diet of very small portions of low-calorie foods. So critical is exercise to caloric balance that at least one exercise physiologist has said, "I'm almost convinced that dieting is totally useless. It's the physical activity aspect of our lifestyle that is the main culprit in our overweight problems."[1]

Not all nutritionists agree. A countervailing school of thought states that so energy efficient are our movements, and so calorically dense our foods, that trying to compensate for overeating through exercise is futile. One pessimistic dietician noted that burning merely one pound of fat requires walking thirty-six miles, or climbing the Washington Monument forty-eight times.[2] More optimistic exercise proponents have suggested an alternate concept of exercise. One must not think of the exercise required to lose weight, they argue, but rather the exercise needed to maintain energy balance daily so that we don't gain weight to begin with. For example, an adult who puts on twelve pounds per year eats about 120 excess calories daily. The exertion required to burn those calories is only a one and a half mile walk, which takes approximately twenty-five minutes at a good clip. The person who can integrate a daily twenty-five-minute walk into her routine, without eating more, will be in energy balance.[3]

We have multiple examples of people who eat highly caloric diets but maintain normal weight simply by virtue of the healthy amount of movement integrated into their lives. Rural Swiss adults, for example, eat about 3,600 calories per day on average, yet are largely slim. While the altitude helps (base metabolism rates rise at higher altitudes), the driving force behind maintaining a healthy weight is their high level of daily activity.[4] Nutrition studies conducted in the 1950s concluded that manual laborers and soldiers in combat could probably consume up to 6,000 calories daily with no adverse effects. Jean Mayer, a prominent American nutritionist in the 1970s and 1980s, wrote about the "busy little nutritionists of the Third Reich" who discovered that they could get almost no productive work out of the slave laborers unless they substantially raised their daily caloric allowance.[5] Manual work simply burns a lot of energy.

Strange as it seems, through the 1940s and 1950s many physicians actually advised *against* exercise for adults, thinking it unnecessary to good health, and possibly even harmful. One physician, Peter Steincrohn, recommended that beyond a round of golf, all else "should be wiped off the slate in the daily schedule of extracurricular exertion."[6] Noting that athletes often had substantially larger hearts than non-athletes, Steincrohn described the syndrome as the potentially fatal "enlarged heart," which should be avoided.[7] Although work at Cambridge University on aging graduates ultimately dispelled the canard, many physicians refused to concede. Noting that non-athletes often lived longer than athletes, one medical advice columnist wrote of weightlifting: "Straining the muscles has been peddled as a cure-all for everything from lumbago to obesity. It usually helps neither, wastes time and energy, and, if overdone, can cause real harm."[8] Steincrohn admonished, "You can be healthy without crooking a little finger in exercise."[9]

However, starting in the 1960s, physicians changed their minds. They did not recommend exercise as an approach to weight control, but many did recommend it as a path to a healthy heart. Nascent understanding of the role of serum cholesterol in arterial plaque buildups impelled many internists and researchers to decide that vigorous exercise, which enlarged the heart and coronary arteries, might make the body more resilient. One cautious physician suggested in 1967 that while exercise might not prevent coronary disease, it might "delay the onset and develop collateral circulation."[10] At the same time, Stanford physicians recruited a broad cohort of male Harvard graduates and tracked them for twenty years. They found that men who expended at least 2,000 calories per week in vigorous exercise had mortality rates one-third to one-quarter lower than their less active classmates.[11] A contemporary study of 18,000 British police officers produced similar results, while the Framingham Heart Study, underway since 1949, concluded the same.[12]

Through the 1980s, more controlled studies that put men on treadmills to measure their heart capacity, tracked their weight and diet, and asked them to keep diaries of daily exertion further validated the theories.[13] Exercise might not make you lighter, but it did produce denser capillary and arterial growth supplying the heart while enlarging the arterial vessels. Contrary to previous thinking, the enlarged vessels and heart chambers were actually less susceptible to infarction, as they allowed more room for blood to pass and provided alternate paths for the blood. In the space of only two decades, conventional wisdom about heart health had been reversed.

What of exercise as a path to controlling obesity? Here the evidence was slower in coming. Much of the early work was done by Jean Mayer in his lab at the Harvard School of Public Health. In studying rats made to do varying amounts of exercise on a wheel, Mayer observed that the rats that ran more simply stayed slimmer, regardless of how much food they were allowed to eat. Follow-up observations on school children found that physically active ones stayed slimmer than their more sedentary classmates, despite actually eating *more* calories each day. Moreover, investigations of workers in a variety of trades found that those who worked manually stayed slimmer, despite (again) eating more than office workers. Meyer concluded wryly that "the ability to sit all day without getting fat has not been bred into the species."[14] Interestingly, the school children professed ignorance about their own level of activity. Girls who stayed motionless 85 percent of the time during a gym volleyball class thought that they moved as much as girls who stayed motionless only 50 percent of the time. One physician could not help expressing his contempt; "Obesity is caused by sloth," he wrote.[15]

The observations collected in the 1960s led to an explosion in the number of adults engaged in physical fitness in the 1970s. Particularly, the fitness "craze" found an outlet in running and also in aerobics classes popularized by Jane Fonda, a notably trim movie star.[16] Jim Fixx wrote multiple articles promoting the "runner's high" through the 1970s, and his *Complete Book of Running* became a bestseller.[17] "There is no doubt that we are in the midst of a fitness explosion," wrote George Leonard, the author of *The Ultimate Athlete*.[18] *Aerobics* by Kenneth Cooper sold over five million copies, while *Total Fitness: In Thirty Minutes a Week* sold half that number. Shops specializing in running shoes sprang up across the country and, notably, a large number of women took up the sport. "I call it my hormonal high," explained one runner in New York City. "But that's only part of the addiction. The running track is my confessional, my wailing wall, my psychiatric couch."[19] Fixx wrote: "Running is the greatest thing that ever happened to me. It gives my life a sense of rhythm. It's not just a game or a sport. It's an adjective—something that defines me."[20]

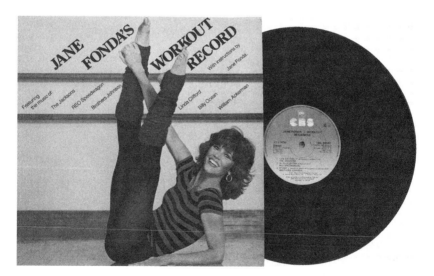

The aerobics craze of groups exercising to music took off in the late 1970s under the tutelage of film star Jane Fonda. Aerobics has morphed to Jazzercise, spin classes, dance aerobics, and competitive yoga, but the social nature of the enterprise has remained constant. *Lynne Sutherland/Alamy Stock Photo*

Other crazes took off at the same time. Isometrics—the periodic tensing of a group of muscles at random times during the day—promised instant and painless fitness. Bicycling drew at least some commuters out of their cars, while more progressive-minded city planners integrated bike lanes into city traffic.[21] Hiking, previously a fringe activity in the United States (though not in the United Kingdom, where it had long attracted a large following) attracted new participants when Colin Fletcher published an inspiring memoir of his hike through the Grand Canyon, *The Man Who Walked Through Time*, following it up with the best-selling how-to guide *The Complete Walker*, which sold nearly half a million copies. The craze produced some awkward culture clashes. One jogger was arrested in Hartford, Connecticut, for "illegal use of the highway by a pedestrian."[22]

Ultimately, however, the fitness craze did not boost participation in athletics substantially across the country. The people who were most likely to turn to jogging, hiking, aerobics, and biking were largely people who were already concerned about health and fitness. Exercise for them was not so much a new phase but rather the next step in a lifetime quest for health. Research in the late 1980s and 1990s bore this out, with most Americans getting exercise merely by "splashing around the local pool" or walking a golf course on the weekends. By 1998, only 40 percent of Americans were getting regular exercise, and half of them admitted that it was not intense.[23] Despite modest improvement in fitness, the trend was passing by most Americans, particularly those who needed exercise the most. "The evidence shows that we are a bunch of fat slobs who do not have activity built into our daily lives," pronounced George Harris, the editor of *American Health*.[24] Most Americans knew, by then, that they *should* be exercising, but still, they could not figure out how to make themselves do it.

DRUGS AND SURGERY

For the many Americans who have found it impossible to comply with diets and lifestyle changes, two artificial boosts have helped some to achieve their goals: drugs and surgery. Both interventions have evolved over the past half-century, to the point where surgical interventions have become highly effective. It is not so with drugs, which tend to produce substantial side effects even while producing only nominal amounts of weight loss. Pharmaceutical companies are still seeking a workable, effective weight-loss drug with few side effects, but as of this writing, they have failed to produce it.

Although people have turned to various folk remedies, foods, and ex-tracts for centuries to burn fat, reduce appetite, and magically melt away pounds, the turn of the twentieth century brought some hope with the use of amphetamines. The best-known amphetamine in the 1940s, Benzedrine, increased alertness, raised blood pressure and pulse rate, increased the sense of "energy," and decreased appetite. People who took Benzedrine tended to find their appetite impaired, though whether the effect was physiological or psychological was initially unclear. That is, it was unclear if amphetamines dulled the appetite, or simply made their users less bored and languid, and thus less interested in eating.[25]

Amphetamines seemed to promise some hope, but early empirical research indicated that the weight loss was less significant than initially hoped for. Only 12 percent of people taking Benzedrine lost substantial weight, and within two years, 98 percent of those who lost weight had gained it back entirely.[26] Moreover, long-term use of amphetamines tended to lead to jitteriness, distraction, and dependency. Weighing their costs against their benefits, amphetamines did not appear promising in achieving long-term weight loss.

Nicotine, a mild stimulant, possessed a similar anorectic effect, and many smokers found that smoking regularly helped them to control their appetites. In 1958, the Cornell Drug Corporation introduced Trims, ciga-rettes laced with tartaric acid, designed specifically to help people with their appetite. The nicotine's anorectic action, coupled with the puckering and drying effect of the tartaric acid, tended to reduce appetite, or at least the appeal of eating. Laboratory tests on Trim run by the Consumers Union failed to produce a more anorectic effect than ordinary cigarettes.[27]

Amphetamines and other stimulants could easily be abused, and anec-dotal reports abounded about young people "strung out" on uppers, unable to concentrate or function normally. Overdoses could prove fatal, as was true with a nineteen-year-old obese boy in 1969 who developed "weak-ness, vomiting, severe hypokalemia (potassium deficiency), and cardiac arrhythmias" on a potent mix of amphetamines, diuretics, and digitalis.[28] However, the greater public health hazard was produced by a mixture of fenfluramine and phentermine, an amphetamine- and serotonin-boosting cocktail. *Fen-phen*, as the compound quickly became known, worked. In an early study, the compound's inventor, Michael Weintraub, found that obese subjects who took it lost an average of thirty-four pounds over seven months.[29] The amphetamine worked its anorectic effect, while the fenfluramine seemed to quell obsessive thoughts about food, probably by raising the level of serotonin in the brain. In 1996, however, researchers concluded that the drug was causing mitral valve dysfunction in nearly a third of the people who took it, leading most doctors to cease prescribing it. In 2005, Wyeth Pharmaceuticals, the manufacturer of the drug, created a $20 billion reserve fund to compensate injured parties.

Other formulations also proved disappointing. Xenical, produced by Roche Pharmaceuticals, induced a seven-pound weight loss over a year, largely by inhibiting the absorption of fat. About two-thirds of people who lost weight on the drug managed to keep it off for a year, but some experienced deficiencies in vitamins D and E, and many experienced pronounced diarrhea—a side effect common to many weight-loss drugs and surgeries. Seven pounds was hardly a panacea for the morbidly obese, but it indicated that the drug might be one of a number of tools in the armament of people grappling with chronic obesity.[30]

The serotonin-boosting effect of the fen part of fen-phen had led drug researchers to experiment with a variety of new drugs with similar actions that might be safer for the heart. Lorcaserin, Contrave, and Qnexa all produced weight loss by targeting various parts of the brain and neurochemical feedback channels. All worked but carried the threat of various side effects, such as anxiety, memory problems, and even suicidal ideation, as had been found with the discontinued drug, Rimonabant. The key seemed to be in mixing the psychoactive drugs in such a way as to produce maximum weight loss at lower doses of each component, thus limiting harmful side effects.[31]

More promising were various surgical remedies, ranging from a gastric sleeve or a lap-band, to a gastric balloon, to the bariatric (intestinal) bypass. All of these techniques physically altered the gut system by either constraining the size of the stomach (via the lap-band and sleeve), artificially filling the stomach (via the balloon), or forcing food to bypass some or nearly all of the gut to limit the body's absorption of calories. The balloon, perhaps the least invasive, involved threading a balloon down the esophagus and inflating it in the stomach, which then limited the patient's stomach capacity. Technically known as the gastric *bubble*, the device was invented by gastroenterologists Lloyd and Mary Garren and approved in 1985. The device worked, insofar as many people with the implant found it easier to control their portions. It was not a cure-all, and it caused ulcers in a few patients, but its ease of insertion, reversibility, and relative safety made it an appealing weight-loss aid.[32]

Gastric stapling was more invasive, involving lessening the size of the stomach by placing surgical staples along a line to reduce its capacity.

The staples were a mechanical fix, forcing the patient to eat less by making overeating very uncomfortable. Although patients reported losing nearly ten pounds a month for the first six months after the procedure, a fair number learned to eat "over" the staples by ingesting large quantities of calories in liquid form. The procedure was fairly simple to perform, taking only about an hour in the operating room, and resulted in few complications.[33]

However, the most successful of the weight-loss surgeries was gastric bypass, in which a large portion of the stomach and small intestine was cut out of the digestion loop by removing a small portion of the stomach from the remainder and attaching it directly to the lower small intestine. The procedure, first performed in 1912 as a jejunostomy, bypassed most of the small intestine where the preponderance of fats were absorbed. A further modification sutured the stomach and upper small intestine back into the small intestine, allowing gastric and pancreatic enzymes to mix with the food and create a more fertile digestive environment. This modified procedure, known as the Roux-en-Y (because of the Y formation of the two channels entering the small intestine) became the standard for weight-loss surgery in the 1990s.

Gastric bypass worked. The majority of patients who underwent the procedure lost substantial amounts of weight and kept off most of it. They experienced few hunger pangs and registered immediate improvement in blood glucose levels, cholesterol, and triglycerides. While the operation was somewhat hazardous—mortality rates were as high as 2 percent for morbidly obese people undergoing the procedure—few patients experienced complications after the procedure.

The exact means by which gastric bypass worked was not entirely clear. In a certain sense, the cure was mechanical; the body simply had fewer feet of bowel in which to absorb fats. However, that did not explain the sharply reduced hunger that most patients experienced immediately. Some researchers hypothesized that in bypassing the stomach, the surgeons had found a critical "off switch" for the body's hunger impulse: a theory given credence with the discovery of the ghrelin-producing cells in the stomach in 2000. Also possible was that hypertrophy of the tissue just around the intestinal suture changed the glucose absorbing properties of the whole gut, leading to different levels of insulin secretion and glucose absorption.[34] Gastric bypass's chief drawback was acute diarrhea; one patient described it as "the most intensive diarrhea imaginable," which may have provided a strong disincentive to eat.[35] One cold-blooded researcher

Roux-en-Y Gastric Bypass (RNY)

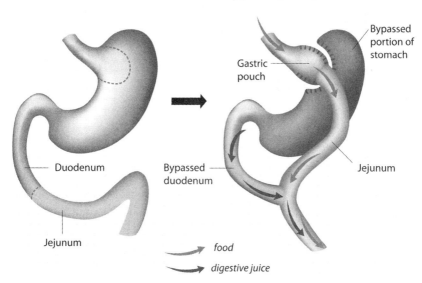

The Roux-en-Y procedure has been the most consistently successful weight-loss surgery. Patients who undergo the procedure find that their hunger cravings abate almost immediately. Most people lose substantial weight, although only a few wind up truly slim. With follow-up therapy, about 80 percent of the patients are able to keep most of the weight off: a portion far more than normal dieters. *Dreamstime Images*

suggested that the "dumping syndrome," characterized by "facial flushing, lightheadedness, palpitations, fatigue, and diarrhea," discouraged patients from eating sugary foods, "contributing to the beneficial effects of the operation."[36]

Physicians have generally reserved gastric bypass for extreme cases of morbid obesity, but as obesity rates have risen and with most Americans finding little success in dieting, exercise, or lifestyle modification, recommendations have changed. The mortality rate from the procedure has declined, and the weight-loss success rate remains high, leading to longer lives. A cheerful study concluded that bariatric surgery led to happier marriages.[37] One gastric surgeon estimated that only about 2 percent of all Americans who could potentially benefit from weight-loss surgery had had it done, a remarkable rate of undertreatment for a proven procedure. In 2013, several physician organizations that were concerned with obesity began to recommend surgical weight-loss procedures for people suffering from "mild to moderate obesity," rather than only for the morbidly obese previously targeted.[38]

A last surgical, or quasi-surgical, procedure that has begun to gain currency in the anti-obesity environment is the fecal transplant. In 2005, scientists at Washington University in St. Louis discovered that a community of bacteria living in the intestines of mice, known as the *biome*, differed substantially depending on whether the mice were thin or fat. Moreover, when scientists took DNA samples of the bacteria living in the mice, they found that gut biomes of thin mice had over 600,000 distinct genes, whereas as the gut biomes of fat mice had fewer than 360,000. The fat mice had lost considerable diversity in their biome, leading scientists to question whether the lost bacteria were responsible for healthy weight maintenance. When they took fecal samples from the lean mice and transplanted them into the intestines of the fat mice, the fat mice lost weight.[39]

This was hardly surprising news to beef farmers, who had long known that introducing antibiotics into cattle feed produced fatter cattle. Martin Blaser, a microbiologist at New York University, taking his lead from the cattle data, proposed that part of the obesity crisis in the United States might be traced to overuse of antibiotics over the previous sixty years. Blaser noted, for example, that aggressive use of antibiotics had largely wiped out the *Helicobacter pylori* strain that caused stomach ulcers. However, the years in which America saw its sharpest decline in stomach ulcers were also the years it saw its sharpest rise in obesity. Perhaps, Blaser reasoned, in the zeal to kill harmful bacteria, American medicine had murdered gut bacteria that guarded against obesity.

Ten years later, Blaser, along with Laura Cox, demonstrated that repeated administration of low-dose penicillin in young infants and young children was highly correlated with the onset of obesity a few years later.[40] (Penicillin used in later years had less of an effect.) Blaser and Cox concluded that the developing human biome, like the developing brain, was particularly susceptible to insults in the early years of life, and once damaged, they might never regain health.[41]

Work by Vanessa Ridaura and colleagues at the same time on human fecal transplants produced similar results.[42] The researchers took fecal samples from sets of twins who were discordant for obesity and implanted the samples into mice guts. Feces from the fat twins produced fat mice, and feces from the thin twins produced thin mice.[43] At nearly the same time, Zhao Lipig, a Chinese microbiologist who had gained substantial amounts of weight on his post-doctoral fellowship in the United States, returned to China determined to lose the flab. Adopting a diet of yam, melon, kale, seaweed, bamboo, and whole grains, he was able to change the balance of bacteria in his gut (which he monitored). In particular, Lipig nurtured the anti-inflammatory *Faecalibacterium prausnitzii* to 14 percent of his gut biome. Within two years, he had lost the weight.[44]

Research on the relationship of the biome to obesity is still new, and much remains to be explored. No researcher is suggesting that gut bacteria, alone, is responsible for obesity. Rather, it appears to be one of several variables, along with diet, sugar, stress, and exercise (or lack thereof) that is contributing to today's epidemic. Healthy gut bacteria ferment plant fiber to create long chain fatty acids that can ultimately be metabolized. These long chain fatty acids are a source of energy but also a potent source of satiation, and thus their absence may be impelling Americans to eat more.

Nobody has conclusively proven that any one calorie is more fattening than another. That is, the old saying that "a calorie is a calorie" still stands. However, we now know that not all calories are equal triggers of satiation. One 500-calorie meal (of processed starches, sugar, and animal fat) hardly touches the satiation switches in the hypothalamus, while another meal, made of fibrous plants, whole grains, and a small amount of protein and fat, digests slowly, leads to the release of leptin and the slow uptake of insulin, and generally leaves the diner feeling calm, full, and satisfied.

Our challenge in this calorie-laden environment is not so much to learn to eat fewer calories, but rather to seek out those calories that will lead to satiation. This involves choosing foods carefully, eating slowly and socially, moving constantly, and avoiding inflammation, stress, and, as we are beginning to understand, superfluous antibiotics.

CHOLESTEROL

One complicating factor in our understanding of diet and obesity has been the confounding variable of cholesterol in the diet and the associated risk of heart disease. Early research on dietary cholesterol in the 1940s showed that a rise in foods that had naturally high levels of cholesterol (notably egg yolks and butterfat) caused at least a temporary rise in cholesterol in the blood.[45] In the early 1950s, researchers observed that fat in the diet could also raise serum cholesterol levels, lending credence to Ancel

Keys's *Seven Countries Study* and his low-fat recommendations. Noboru Kimura's early study into the low rate of heart disease among Japanese men further confirmed the idea. After surveying medical records for 10,000 men and autopsying over 1,000 hearts, Kimura concluded that the culprit was fat. Japanese men suffered heart disease at only one-tenth the rate of American men, and they got about ten percent of their daily calories from fat. Americans, meanwhile, consumed 40 percent of their calories through fat. Comparative studies of diets and heart disease in Bantu, colored, and white men in Cape Town, South Africa, and of Italian men living in (low-fat) Naples and (high-fat) Bologna seemed to offer incontrovertible proof that fat killed.[46]

Cholesterol, however, is not fat. A modified steroid (technically a *sterol*) produced by all animals, the molecule is an essential component of cell membranes and of particular importance in building neural tissue. Only a small portion of all the body's cholesterol is ingested in the diet; most of it is manufactured. Further complicating matters, most animals are able to regulate their production of cholesterol in response to dietary levels, producing more or less as needed. Humans possess only an imperfect hemostatic control mechanism; only the liver is capable of adjusting its cholesterol production.

Virtually all of the early evidence linking fat with cholesterol was observational and statistical; people who ate a lot of fat appeared to have high levels of *serum* cholesterol (that is, cholesterol dissolved in the blood), and populations that consumed a lot of animal fat seemed to die of coronary disease more frequently. After death, autopsies of heart attack sufferers exposed thick arterial plaques of cholesterol.

Fat people do not necessarily have higher cholesterol, however. One study published in 1959 showed little correlation between obesity and cholesterol, suggesting that while fat in a diet raised cholesterol levels, fat in the body did not.[47] At about the same time, Frederick Stare observed that people eating low-fat diets showed lower levels of serum cholesterol and associated "fat protein particles" (known today as *lipoproteins*) regardless of how much cholesterol they ate. That is, egg yolks without fat did not seem nearly as harmful as a slab of butter.[48] Researchers were able to make many relevant observations but could not produce a coherent model of diet and heart health.

Within a few years, however, the landscape changed. Food science researchers at the University of California's agricultural campus in Davis noted that while butter raised serum cholesterol, butter mixed with soy oil lowered it. Similarly, animals fed lard in their feed showed high levels of serum cholesterol, while those fed a modified diet containing the same amount of fat but sourced from cottonseed oil had low levels. Even more interesting was that monkeys fed raw corn oil showed low levels of cholesterol, but monkeys fed corn oil that had been *hydrogenated*—that is, transformed to a room-temperature solid fat by having hydrogen bubbled through it—had high levels.[49] It seemed that all fat was not the same. Animal fats increased cholesterol while plant fats lowered it, except for plant fats that were solid at room temperature, which tended to raise it.[50]

Things got even more complicated a decade later when researchers observed that some liquid plant oils seemed to have cholesterol-raising properties after they had been heated to high temperatures. By the early 1970s, researchers proposed that the relationship between fats and cholesterol was complex. Fats could transport cholesterol in and out of cells, and polyunsaturated (liquid plant oils) were able to effectively dissolve cholesterol, while saturated (animal) fats not only could not, they appeared to actually block the clearing action of the unsaturated fats.[51] Moreover, people who stayed slim and physically active seemed better able to thwart the destructive effect of saturated fat, most likely by creating more robust arterial networks in their hearts. This seemed to solve the Swiss paradox: the low rates of heart disease among Swiss farmers who ingested nearly 50 percent of the calories from saturated animal fats.

By the early 1990s, scientists spoke of "good" fats (olive, safflower, and nut oils) and "bad" fats (lard, butter, beef tallow, and palm and coconut oil). Not only were the good fats not harmful, they were actually helpful. Nutritionists began to push their high-risk patients to Mediterranean diets, which are rich in olive oil and touted for their protective benefits.[52] Meats, by contrast, appeared dangerous. Even longtime beef lovers began to question their dietary mix. Sales of beef fell in the 1990s, while sales of chicken rose. Most momentously, McDonald's, for the first time, offered a low-fat hamburger entree—the McLean Deluxe—consisting of a beef patty diluted with carrageenan.[53]

By the 2000s, American had grown fairly sophisticated in differentiating good fat from bad fat, "good" (HDL) cholesterol from "bad" (LDL) cholesterol, and *cis* fats from *trans* fats. More than a few Americans migrated to vegetarian or modified vegetarian diets, limiting red meat in their diets and substituting fish and poultry. Hardcore health nuts turned to vegan diets, which contained no animal products. After undergoing bypass surgery, President Bill Clinton turned to a diet heavy on legumes, fruits, vegetables, and almond milk, shunning carbohydrates of all sorts and animal protein. The humble bean became the "glory child" of the vegan age, appearing in recipes ranging from veggie burgers to bean-based pasta sauces and stir-fried tofu.[54] A small portion of the population, residing largely in upscale professional neighborhoods in the coastal cities, was growing thinner and healthier, even as most of the country was becoming sicker and fatter.

9

Self-Control

REINING IN THE IMPULSE

Staying thin should be easy: just eat less. However, when appealing food is easily available, eating less means constantly resisting desire, and this is very, very hard. Resisting desire is so hard, and so exhausting, that it has given rise to entirely new fields of study in both psychology and behavioral economics.

In a series of experiments with preschool-aged children in the early 1960s, researchers rated them on *impulse control*. In the most famous study, a psychologist left a child in a room sitting at a table with a marshmallow in the middle. The child was instructed that he was allowed to eat the marshmallow, but if he waited until the psychologist returned (about fifteen minutes), he could have two marshmallows. That is, the child's ability to delay gratification would yield greater long-term rewards. Some of the children were able to wait for the researcher's return, and some were not.

In subsequent years, the children who had been able to withstand the call of the marshmallow showed striking differences from the children who had not been able to resist. At age fourteen, they demonstrated higher levels of social and academic competence. They were better able to deal with frustration. They had longer concentration spans, performed better in school, used language at a higher level, and displayed substantially higher levels of executive functioning. That is, even in early adolescence, they were better able to plan for the future, make and achieve long-term goals, and effectively weigh priorities. They were deemed by parents and teachers to be more mature and more confident. Four years later, these same marshmallow resisters scored higher on their SATs.

Even more surprising was that there were differences in the children who had succumbed to the lure of the marshmallow. Researchers had timed how long it took kids to eat the marshmallow. Fourteen years later, researchers discovered a strong relationship between the length of time that the kids had waited to eat the marshmallow and their SAT scores.[1]

Later in life, the marshmallow resisters demonstrated greater success in nearly everything they attempted. They graduated from college in higher numbers, earned more money, and gained more promotions. They stayed married longer, committed fewer crimes, maintained more friendships, and stayed healthier. Although it is too soon to really know, it appears that they will live longer. Self-control is hardwired in the brain; some people simply have more of it than others. The initial set-point appears to be consistent through life and (soberingly) is highly predictive of success along multiple axes of achievement.

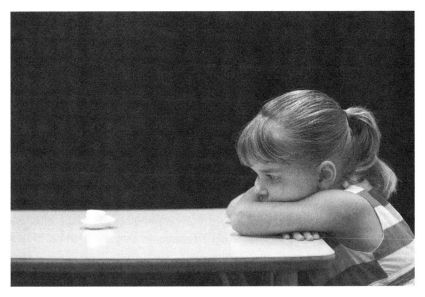

The marshmallow experiment: Kids who are able to resist eating the marshmallow for about fifteen minutes while the researcher leaves the room show a higher degree of impulse control throughout their lives. *University of Rochester Archives*

As relates to obesity, self-control interests us because it would seem to be the precise component we lack when we gain weight. If we could all simply resist the siren call of food, none of us would be fat. However, this cannot be entirely true, as there is little evidence that the raw amount of self-control in society has diminished in the last half-century, yet we are all much fatter. Something else has changed.

Recent research has forced us to modify our understanding of self-control. While it is true that people have relatively different amounts of self-control from birth, in any one person the ability to control one's impulses—to act with *volition*—varies over the course of a year, or even a day. Acting with volition can be termed willpower, the conscious steering of one's life. Willpower is expressed in making decisions, evaluating trade-offs, prioritizing tasks, and following through on those priorities. It is the difference between simply following a well-trodden path along with the rest of a group and consciously turning off of that path to take yourself to a preferred destination.

We can model self-control in three different ways: as a *skill*, as a *knowledge-base*, or as a *task*. If self-control is a skill, then we might expect that people could practice and get better at it. While there is some evidence that this is true, for the most part (as demonstrated by the marshmallow experiment), self-control is constant from a young age. As for the second model, people with greater impulse control don't really have to learn it; they just *have* it. If self-control is knowledge-based, then it might be something that could be taught formally, the way we teach any other skill in a vocational class. Moreover, while intense therapy can help impulsive people become slightly more thoughtful in their decision-making, they really never get good at it. Impulsive people generally *know* that they are acting impulsively, but they do so regardless. The problem is not one of ignorance.

Several compelling new analyses point to the third model as the most likely: self-control as a task. To take a recent influential experiment, Jonathan Levav and Shai Danziger observed the behavior of parole boards in Israel. The work of a parole board is to decide whether a prisoner's exemplary behavior justifies an early release from prison. The risk is that too early a release places society in danger, and thus the default decision (that is, the *safe* path) is to deny parole. Levav and Danziger found a striking correlation between the conclusion of the parole board and the time of day at which it heard a particular case. Prisoners judged early in the morning, or shortly after lunch, when the judges were well-rested and, more importantly, well-fed, were far more likely to be released. Prisoners coming before the board later in the morning or afternoon, when the judges were tired and hungry, were one-seventh as likely to be paroled. The difference was so stark as to nearly dictate the decision merely by the luck of the schedule.[2]

What Levav and Danziger had observed was *decision-fatigue*, more technically called *ego depletion*.[3] Even good decision-makers only have so much capacity for exerting willful control over their thought processes and for reining in their own impulses. Individuals subjected to a series of difficult trade-offs soon grow exhausted and resort to default or safe thinking. Whether customizing a car you are ordering (What kind of wheels? Standard engine or turbo-charged? Leather or cloth?), registering for wedding gifts, speccing out a personal computer, or planning a party, everybody invests more in the initial choices than in the later ones. The ability to make thoughtful choices is finite; we all quickly grow exhausted and fall back on non-thoughtful options, whether suggested by a sales associate, a financial planner, or a computer algorithm. When really exhausted, we choose to simply *not* choose, and we put off decision-making until the next day. That is essentially what the parole boards were doing late in the day. Unable to summon the mental energy to rigorously evaluate the risk that a given prisoner posed to society, they threw the prisoner back in jail knowing that he would not do any harm there.

Willpower can be depleted in numerous ways. People subjected to difficult tasks, emotional turmoil, or even physically strenuous challenges all give up more quickly when confronted shortly after with difficult puzzles. One group of research subjects was placed in front of dishes of chocolate chip cookies and radishes—half the group was allowed to eat the cookies; the other half could only eat the radishes. The radish-eating group gave up on a set of anagram puzzles substantially quicker than the cookie-eating group. In a similar experiment, subjects forced to watch the emotionally charged movie *Terms of Endearment* (in which the protagonist dies of cancer) while being asked to suppress their emotions also gave up more quickly on a puzzle. And in a classic challenge of volitional thinking, a group of subjects shown a series of slides with names of colors written on them ("red," "blue," "yellow," or "green") but printed out in a mismatched color, had to correctly identify the color of the typeface— that is, they had to override their impulse to simply read the word. All took progressively more time to accomplish this as the experiment went on. They simply grew exhausted.[4]

Willpower appears to be a limited resource and expending it on volitional thinking and resisting impulses exhausts it. The limitation is not simply psychological. People consume substantial energy thinking analytically about difficult ideas or resisting desires, actually depleting the glucose in their brains. It is one of the reasons that people do not think clearly when hungry (their brains are literally starving), and it is also one of the confounding paradoxes of dieting—we are asked to resist the impulse of indulging in food when our brains are particularly ill-equipped to resist an impulse. One of the foremost researchers on ego depletion, Roy Baumeister, notes that willpower is "more than a metaphor."[5]

As our willpower is depleted and as our brain glucose level drops, our thinking processes change. We become impatient and irritable. Pleasure beckons us more intensely, and we are more likely to succumb to temptation. (Few people wake up fresh in the morning planning on violating their marriage vows or drinking too much.) To a large degree, when our brains are tired, we choose not to choose by avoiding trade-offs, putting off major decisions, and becoming (in the words of science writer John Tierney) "cognitive misers."[6]

Good decision-makers are born with a great ability to delay gratification, but they also adopt a life strategy of making as few decisions as possible. That is, they develop good daily habits that preclude the need to make decisions. If you sign up to exercise with a group at the same time every day, then you wind up doing it automatically—you don't have to think about the trade-off of exercising versus not exercising. Similarly, eating the same breakfast and lunch every day, wearing the same clothes, and following the same daily habits all preserve cogitative energy for more important and difficult decisions that come up during the course of the day. Corporate executives wear pretty boring attire because it's the uniform of the job, but also in part because they have more important decisions to think about than their clothes. If you are spending a good deal of time every morning thinking about your outfit, you are starting the day already mentally depleted.

Ego depletion also helps explain some of the bad decisions that poor people make. People are poor, in part, because they have not made good life decisions (dropping out of school, committing crimes, having children too young, etc.), but also in part they make bad choices because they are poor and thus exhausted. Lacking money, poor people are forced to consider many more daily trade-offs than are rich people—Walk or ride? Buy the branded soap or the generic? Take advantage of the sale on shoes or save the money for a trip? By the time they get to the supermarket, poor people have far less energy to resist the pull of candy bars and soda than do wealthier people who have hoarded their mental energy during the day. Similarly, forcing yourself to go to the gym, which requires overriding the impulse to be slothful, is easier when you still have a healthy supply of willpower stored up. The end of a stressful day is no time to force yourself to take on difficult and unpleasant tasks.

Our obesogenic environment depletes our willpower constantly by forcing us to expend energy resisting tasty food. One of the most successful strategies to staying thin relies not so much on resisting temptation but rather on removing it. Thin people like cookies and ice cream too, but they are less likely to allow these products into their homes, offices, and schools, and thus they do not expend energy resisting them. Similarly, removing fast-food restaurants, candy machines, convenience stores, and donut shops from our environment does not mean that we never indulge, but rather that on a daily basis, we expend less mental energy thinking about not indulging.[7] We achieve similar effects by removing coffee-and-cookie platters and candy bowls from our offices, as well as the ubiquitous leftovers placed in conference rooms after every corporate lunch.[8]

ENVIRONMENTAL CUES

In 1968, Stanley Schachter, a professor of psychiatry at Columbia University, observed differential eating habits of obese and normal-weight subjects. Under the guise of a "taste test," he had subjects come to his lab having skipped the previous two meals. Half of the subjects were then allowed to fill up on a buffet of sandwiches while others were kept hungry. They were then placed in front of several bowls of different kinds of crackers and asked to eat as many of them as they wished and record the taste sensations.

Unbeknownst to the volunteers, the experiment was not really about tasting; it was rather an effort to observe if heavy and normal-weight subjects adjusted their eating depending on whether or not they had just filled up at the buffet. The researchers were simply counting the number of crackers that the subjects ate. As expected, the normal-weight subjects modulated their intake depending on whether they had just filled up at the buffet. The hungry volunteers ate more crackers; the full volunteers ate fewer. However, for the obese volunteers, the meal at the buffet had little effect on the number of crackers they ate. They modulated their intake not based on how hungry they were, but rather on how tasty they rated the crackers. Insensitive to their own internal hunger cues, they ate in response to the external food environment.[9] Schachter wrote that the obese subjects "literally do not know when they are physiologically hungry."[10]

In a follow-up experiment, Schachter placed subjects on a very bland diet akin to the liquid protein that would be introduced as a dieting aid a decade later. That is, the diet assuaged hunger pangs and provided nutrition, but it was in no way appetizing or alluring. Thin subjects drank more of the protein when they were hungry and less when they were not, unconsciously adjusting their food intake to comport with internal hunger cues. By contrast, obese subjects drank almost none of the stuff, even if they had not eaten for hours or days. They were unwilling to ingest nutrition that was not appetizing, even when their empty stomachs might have signaled an urge to eat. Again, the perception of *hunger* seemed to be significantly different between heavy and normal-weight subjects, with the heavy subjects more susceptible to external food cues and less sensitive to internal hunger cues. Writing about this phenomenon a few years later, Richard Spark, a professor of medicine at Harvard, deemed obese people "exquisitely responsive" to a variety of external food cues.[11]

Further studies confirmed the observation. Obese people were more likely to eat at a certain time of day regardless of how frequently they had consumed, even when clocks were deliberately mis-set by an hour or more. They were more likely to enter food stores with appetizing wares regardless of their objective hunger states, in contrast to thinner subjects who ignored the displays when they had eaten recently. And they were more likely to indulge in tasty snacks even if a formal meal was imminent, in contrast to thinner people who resisted the snacks for fear of ruining their appetites.[12]

Such experiments give us some insight as to why it is so difficult for many people to resist eating in the obesogenic environment in which we find ourselves. For people who look to external stimuli for guidance in eating, the world has become a toxic environment, saturated with stimulus that requires near-superhuman qualities to resist. Given our greater insight today about the limits of human resistance (the ego depletion discussed earlier), we cannot be surprised at the epidemic of obesity in which we find ourselves.

Newer research supports the disconnect of eating from objective hunger for many people. Brian Wansink, a food psychologist at Cornell, has conducted extensive research on cues that trigger eating and overeating in many people. His findings suggest that people who are sensitive to external cues rather than internal ones eat more or less depending on the size and color of their plates, the volume of background music and intensity of lighting in a restaurant, the physical location of their table in the restaurant (people sitting near front windows are less likely to order dessert), and whether they use chopsticks or forks (chopstick users at Chinese restaurants eat less). Many of Wansink's findings are surprising, or at least counterintuitive. For example, when faced with a can of stacked Pringles potato chips, people will eat fewer if every seventh chip is dyed with red food coloring. (The odd-colored chips resulted in people eating 50 percent fewer.)

Some of Wansink's observations are more intuitive. People are likely to eat less if they leave food on the stove rather than in large serving dishes brought to the table. They eat less if food is stored out of sight in cabinets rather than lined up on countertops. They eat less if kitchen cabinet doors are opaque rather than transparent. They drink less wine if they pour it into tall, thin glasses rather than short, wide ones. It seems that for many people, eating is a response to practically every facet of their environment *except* the actual quantity of food in their stomachs.[13]

Given that many people find external cues powerful inducements to eat, and given, also, that we are now subjected to endless cues during the course of our days that quickly exhaust our ability to resist, is there any hope for the obese? Certainly, obese people achieve good results when they place themselves in a highly restrictive environment—a Marine boot camp or a residential health spa. However, at least some obese people have been able to lose weight after having undergone intensive behavioral therapy in an effort to retrain themselves to respond less intensely to environmental cues.

Obese people who undergo "intensive" lifestyle retraining therapy do lose weight and manage to keep it off for significant lengths of time.[14] Starting in the early 1970s and under the guidance of Albert Stunkard of the University of Pennsylvania, university-affiliated hospitals at several medical schools established weight-loss clinics that relied on long-term behavioral counseling.[15] Patients were taught to recognize cues and situations that were likely to get them to eat, and they were given coping mechanisms to avoid those situations or to better resist them.[16] Treatments included group therapy, individual counseling, videotapes, and peer support groups. For most of these programs, clinicians found that "more was more"; that is, the more intensively immersed the patients were in behavior-changing therapy, the more weight they were able to lose and keep off.

Success with behavioral therapy suggests the essential soundness of the approach of TOPS and Weight Watchers, as discussed in Chapter 8. Both of these programs (Weight Watchers, in particular) rely on helping people to identify the environmental cues that stimulate their appetites and to learn how to avoid those cues, or at least temporarily resist them until they can safely distance themselves.[17] The problem, of course, is that Weight Watchers, and all behavioral therapy, is hard, slow, and frequently expensive. For the millions of obese Americans seeking a quick and easy fix to their weight problem, research suggests that they are searching in vain. *Eating* differently presupposes *living* differently, which requires a commitment to examining every aspect of the way people construct their lives. Losing weight is not to be pursued flippantly.

SOCIAL CUES

Constructing an environment conducive to staying slim requires social structures as well. Humans, the most intensely social of all animals, constantly look to each other for cues on a wide variety of behaviors, beliefs, habits, and thought patterns. People look to their social peers for inspiration and guidance on such diverse attributes as syntax, religion, politics, professional goals, and fashion. To an extraordinary degree, people recapitulate the habits of tribe and clan in their family choices, daily patterns, and eating and exercise habits.

One great problem with obesity is that it tends to isolate its sufferers, cutting them off from precisely the sorts of supportive relationships and intimate reinforcement that they need to be able to substitute for the gratification of food. "Obesity discourages the obese," wrote one researcher in 1968, by which he meant that the state of being obese is self-reinforcing.[18] Recent research on addiction validates the point. Addicts learn, at an early age, to use drugs for solace and pleasure rather than turn to social engagement for these experiences. If food can be thought of like a drug, then overeating is, in part, a maladaptive strategy for garnering pleasure when more healthy avenues, such as social engagement or satisfying pursuits, are unavailable. One recovered addict wrote in 2016, "the circuitry that normally connects us to one another socially has been channeled instead into drug seeking. To return our brains to normal, then, we need more love, not more pain."[19]

In 1976, Kelly Brownell, later a celebrated obesity researcher but at the time a graduate student in psychology at Rutgers, became curious about weight loss. Thinking that eating habits might be influenced by social cues, he enlisted twenty-nine married obese people interested in losing weight and placed them into three groups. In the first group, spouses were recruited as trained active cooperators in the weight-loss program; in the second, the spouses were supportive but untrained; and in the third, spouses were actively hostile to the weight-loss enterprise. After eight months, volunteers in the first group, with the supportive and trained spouses, had lost thirty pounds on average versus only fifteen pounds for volunteers in the other two groups.

Brownell used his findings to develop a new weight-loss program called LEARN (Lifestyle, Exercise, Attitudes, Relationships, Nutrition) with an accompanying textbook and support groups. In the midst of the Atkins low-carbohydrate craze, LEARN espoused a more comprehensive change in life habits with the idea of helping people not so much lose weight as permanently change the way they lived, and so allow them to eat and move differently.[20]

Brownell refined his ideas behind weight loss and weight maintenance over the following decades, always cleaving to the idea that living thin entailed a comprehensive commitment to habits of thinness—daily structures and schedules and habits of exercise —but a critical component of Brownell's insight remained that eating and moving were fundamentally social activities, and thus were highly susceptible to social suggestion. In fact, the essential prerequisite to weight loss and weight maintenance—motivation—was itself largely a result of social pressure. Thin people stayed thin because of social pressure to stay thin and social validation for being thin. Commitment, always flagging, could be bolstered by friends, associates, relatives, and peers. Beyond carbohydrates, sugar, fat, exercise, portion control, and fiber lay the essential motivation to stick to a thin lifestyle. "In my mind," admitted Brownell in 2003, "the most important thing in weight loss is motivation."[21]

Other scholarship bore out the claim. As far back as 1974, George Mann postulated that diets were worthless, as the dieters always gained the weight back. Rather, the only true hope for the obese lay in group therapy and behavior modification. That is, fat people needed to relearn how to live life more comprehensively and always live within a social context. Slim people stayed slim because they lived slim lives, not because they simply ate better.[22] Not surprisingly, a series of studies on the long-term efficacy of weight-loss programs conducted in the early 2000s found that only two, TOPS and Weight Watchers, consistently produced long-term sustainable weight loss. Those programs were the two that required the greatest amount of social engagement in the weight-loss program from their adherents.[23]

A great deal of empirical and anecdotal evidence bore out the critical role of social pressure in maintaining weight loss. The high levels of success garnered by fat camps and residential weight-loss clinics spoke to both environmental and social factors, as did the French habit of always eating socially at structured mealtimes.[24] Various studies of social networks found that thin women, in particular, tended to actively seek out other thin women as friends and colleagues: in part to maintain social status, but also in part to facilitate their own efforts to maintain a lower weight.[25]

Exercise, too, was socially impelled. While some people were naturally more athletically inclined than others, the social dynamic of team sports seemed to be particularly important in imbuing individuals with regular habits of exercise. One study found that young people who had engaged in organized team sports were two to three times more likely to continue to participate in athletics as adults than others who had been athletically vigorous as youngsters but had exercised alone.[26] That is, simply being athletically inclined as a child did not produce a lifetime of fitness, but being socially engaged while pursuing athletics did. The authors of the study, interested (like Brownell) in the genesis of motivation, admitted that psychological barriers to exercise were profound and complex; many people just lacked the "self-regulatory skills necessary to engage in the complex sets of behaviors referred to as exercise habits."[27] Social engagement with other exercisers catalyzed the decision; it was simply much easier to get yourself to the gym when all of your friends were going.

The social model of fitness and healthy eating further validated the observations of many researchers that people stayed thin when they lived in an environment that enforced thinness, and that most people got fat when they lived in an environment that allowed them to do so. People simply had far less control over their eating and movement than they supposed, and maintaining motivation in the absence of social cues was unrealistic for most. Amish children, wealthy society women, aboriginal tribesmen, and native Inuit all stayed thin because they *lived* thin, as did virtually everybody around them. If you removed the environmental and social framework around them and plunged them into an obesogenic environment, few would have the motivation to remain that way.

PRICING CUES

People are not only getting fatter because food is more available, but also because it is very cheap. Carbohydrates, the cheapest form of calories, are so inexpensive as to be easily affordable for even the poorest Americans. A 2,000-calorie loaf of bread may retail for as little as 89 cents. A three-liter bottle of store-brand soda, with 1,200 calories, usually retails for under $2. And a package of store-brand macaroni and cheese, containing 1,400 calories, retails for under a dollar.

The poorest Americans, who also happen to be the fattest, tend to be quite sensitive to price increases. One easy way to change our food environment is simply to raise the price of food. Although grocers and food producers are loathe to do this for fear of losing market share, research in manipulating prices has demonstrated that even modest price hikes produce significant swings in buying habits. In Minnesota, for example, a group of researchers halved the prices of items in a vending machine that contained less than three grams of fat—baked potato chips, for example, and pretzels—while holding the prices of other items constant. Over three weeks, sales of the low-fat items rose by 80 percent. Performing a similar experiment in two school cafeterias, the researchers halved the price of bags of carrots and cut-up fruit. In the wealthier of the two schools, sales of carrots and fruit doubled; in the poorer of the two schools, sales quadrupled.[28] People may have food preferences, but those preferences are often overridden by considerations of price.

If grocers are unwilling to raise prices on non-nutritional food, perhaps the government can do it for them by imposing a junk-food tax. Kelly Brownell and Michael Jacobson proposed a national 1 cent soda tax in the late 1990s to no avail, but similar taxes elsewhere have succeeded in reducing the consumption of sugared drinks.[29] In Brazil, for example, a 1 percent increase in the cost of sugar-sweetened drinks led to nearly a 1 percent decline in consumption (poor people cut back more than rich people).[30] A more limited effort at the cafeteria of the Brigham and Women's Hospital in Boston produced similar results; a temporary 35-percent price increase on sugared drinks led to a 26-percent decline in consumption.[31] One group of nutrition researchers hoping to reduce the nearly insatiable demand for sugary drinks in India estimated that a 20-percent tax on sugared drinks in that country could reduce the nation's obese population by 11.2 million over a decade and prevent 400,000 cases of type II diabetes.[32]

Savings in lost productivity and reduced demand for medical care could total $10 billion or more.

Michael Bloomberg, the mayor of New York City from 2002 until 2014, attempted a different approach to modifying the food environment when he asked the city's Board of Public Health to prohibit the sale of sugared drinks in restaurants in sizes greater than sixteen ounces. Bloomberg justified the effort by saying, "I've got to defend my children, and yours, and do what's right to save lives. Obesity kills."[33] Although the rule was ultimately nullified by the courts (the judge ruled that an administrative agency did not have the power to prohibit the sale of a legal product), the effort stood on firm empirical ground.[34] While the American Beverage Association rejected the effort, claiming that "150 years of research finds that people consume what they want," behavioral research had demonstrated that people were highly susceptible to portion, container, and plate size in modifying their consumption of food and drink.[35] Future efforts along these lines will need to establish that food is toxic in certain quantities, and thus it ought to be a candidate for regulation in the same way as alcohol.

An additional possibility for modifying the food environment would be to standardize portion sizes across the restaurant and prepared-food industries, so that a single serving of a particular dish (apple pie, steak, hamburger, nachos, etc.) would have to comport to a standard size. At present, Americans are inept at estimating the calories in a given restaurant portion. One study showed that restaurant patrons underestimated the calorie count of a variety of dishes by nearly half and the fat content by more than half.[36]

Given the limited ability of most people to exercise control over their impulse to eat, a long-term response to obesity must be to change the food environment so that we are not forced to constantly resist temptation. We can choose to regulate how and where food is sold, how and where it can be consumed, how food is priced, or how food is presented. Any of these changes in the environment promise to lower food consumption and reduce obesity. All will be opposed by the food and restaurant industries, as well as by retailers, much as restrictions on tobacco were opposed by tobacco companies a generation ago. However, once we accept that we are quite literally eating ourselves to death and are largely incapable of controlling our own impulse to eat, we can exercise the administrative power of the state to change our environment and save at least a few lives.

10

Disparate Impacts

ETHNIC AND RACIAL DIFFERENCES

Obesity does not attack with equal force everywhere. As I've discussed in earlier chapters, the poor population suffers particularly from the effects of an obesogenic environment, as do people living at lower altitudes and in colder climates. It helps to live in a walkable neighborhood where sunny weather induces you to get out and move.[1] It helps to live near highly paid and highly educated neighbors and to socialize, work, and lunch with those who live low-stress lives. Moreover, in the United States, it helps, too, to be White or Asian.[2]

Obesity disproportionately hits Latin Americans, African Americans, and Native Americans. The adult obesity rate in those groups hovers at, respectively, 50, 50, and 70 percent, versus about 33 percent for adult Caucasians.[3] Rates vary around the country and by income, but even in the same city and at the same income level, the racial disparities are significant. One study of ethnic neighborhoods around Chicago found childhood obesity rates of 12 percent in a middle-class White neighborhood, 34 percent in a Mexican neighborhood, and 56 percent in a Black neighborhood.[4]

Almost all people get fatter when they move to the United States. Mexicans are fairly obese these days, but they get more so once they emigrate.[5] By contrast, immigrants from Asian countries (particularly China and Japan) tend to start out thin, but they, too, get heavier as they stay in the United States longer. In Hawaii, people of Japanese extraction are thinner

139

than people of European or native Hawaiian ancestry, but they are fatter than their relatives who stayed in Japan.[6] When they move to the mainland United States, they get fatter still. Chinese immigrants, who long resisted American dietary patterns, are also falling victim to hyper-palatable processed foods. Jennifer Tang, a first-generation Chinese American, notes that although she is a rarity—a "full-figured Chinese female"—she is merely a harbinger of a coming trend. "Thanks to the globalization of fast food," she writes, "I know I won't be unique for long."[7]

African Americans have been particularly susceptible to obesity, in part due to lower incomes, but also due to different dietary and cultural norms. At age ten, Black girls are eleven pounds heavier than White girls, while their mothers are seventeen and a half pounds heavier than White mothers.[8] The last half-century has been particularly difficult for Black children; the obesity rate in Black teenage boys jumped from 2 to 13 percent in the three decades after 1963 and in Black teenage girls from 5 to 16 percent during the same period.[9]

Poverty is clearly part of the driver. Middle-class Black women who grew up poor are twice as likely to be obese as adults as middle-class Black women who grew up middle-class, suggesting that eating patterns established in youth are hard to shed.[10] However, there is more than poverty at play. In part, Black women may be heavier because they pay a

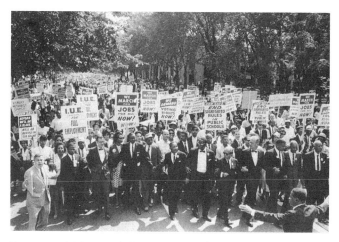

The current high rate of obesity among African Americans is relatively recent, as photos of civil rights demonstrators in the 1960s shows. *Getty Images*

lower social cost for being fat than do White women. A team of researchers from Stony Brook University (SUNY) interviewed nearly 6,000 White and Black teenage girls and found that while all overweight and obese adolescent girls pay a penalty in perceptions of attractiveness, Black overweight girls face "a significantly smaller penalty."[11]

In part, African Americans are heavier because their diet reflects the norms of the poor Southern communities where many lived until two generations ago; White Americans are also heavier from the same region. But in part, African Americans are heavier because of the greater amount of accumulated stress in their lives. One research team identified the "anticipatory stress" or "racism-related vigilance" that permeates the psyches of many African Americans. Studying 3,100 Chicagoans of various races, the researchers found that Whites lived with little of this type of stress, while Blacks lived with a great deal of it. Asking such questions as, "In your day-to-day life, how often do you: 1) Try to prepare for possible insults from other people before leaving home? 2) Feel that you always have to be very careful about your appearance to get good service or avoid being harassed? and 3) Try to avoid certain social situations and places?" researchers found that on a 7-point scale, Blacks averaged hypertensive responses of 3.8, Latinos 2.5, and Whites 1.8. Given that stress, and its concomitant rise in cortisol levels, is highly correlated with obesity, we must ascribe at least part of the racially disparate obesity levels in the United States to racism, or fear of its effects.[12]

The racial obesity effect spills over to nearby neighbors, confirming the many observations that obesity is somewhat contagious. Studies of residents of predominantly White, Hispanic, and Black neighborhoods found that they were thinner or fatter based on the race of their neighbors, irrespective of their own race and income.[13] All of these observations confirm my earlier discussion about environment: few people can escape the food effects of the environment in which they live, whether that environment is racially, geographically, or economically defined. When Black people leave Black neighborhoods and move to White ones, they tend to start eating Whiter, just as poor people moving to wealthier neighborhoods start eating wealthier.[14] We shouldn't be surprised. When Americans are relocated abroad because of corporate transfers, they tend to start eating as natives, except for soldiers on active duty who eat American food on base and get fat like Americans. More than a few children of American servicemen raised in Germany tell of childhoods eating imported sugared cereals and going out to the local McDonald's franchise on base.

DIFFERENCES AROUND THE WORLD

Although this book concentrates on obesity in the United States, it is worth digressing to examine differential obesity rates around the world as we look at rates at home. Obesity is hardly confined to the United States. Over a billion people worldwide are overweight or obese, and the number is rising rapidly nearly everywhere. Nonetheless, obesity is becoming concentrated in the poorer nations of the world, particularly in Polynesia, Southeast Asia, Latin America, China, and India. While it is true that the poorest people in the poorest countries (mainly in sub-Saharan Africa) remain thin and frequently undernourished, poor people in middle-income and developing countries are growing obese. In particular, as Western restaurants, processed foods, and snacking habits invade developing nations, and as populations have greater access to motorized vehicles, obesity rates increase. For illustration's sake, about one billion people worldwide suffered from hypertension in 2000; by 2025, the number will be over one and a half billion. Nearly all of the growth is taking place in the world's poorer nations.[15]

The culprits are the usual: sugar, fats, processed foods, sedentary lives, and television. What is odd about the obesity epidemic in poorer countries is how rapidly it is developing. As recently as 1989, only 10 percent of Mexicans were overweight or obese. Today, the country is fatter than the United States. In Mexico, Colombia, Turkey, South Africa, and Jordan, more than half of the rural women are overweight. In China, daily consumption of fat has doubled in a generation, and more than half the population now suffers from hypertension. Mexicans now consume more sugared sodas than do Americans.[16]

Worldwide, obesity is growing because people are getting wealthier, but also because food is getting cheaper. The price of beef in constant dollars has dropped by nearly two-thirds since 1970, even as per capita incomes have grown (in real dollars) in most countries. At the same time, added income has allowed a rapidly growing middle class to move less. Half of all Chinese households now own a television. The fastest growing auto markets in the world are in China and India.

As with the United States, worldwide obesity is an artifact of genes meeting a changing environment. Some ethnic groups are genetically programmed to get fat as soon as extra calories are available. Samoans, the fattest people on Earth today, seem to suffer from an extreme version of a thrifty gene wherein their satiation response seems weak if not entirely absent. In the past, food shortages and physically demanding toil kept their weight in check. Westernization and mechanization have both created a health crisis for the group, present on their native islands and in immigrant groups in the United States.[17] Certain subpopulations in the Indian subcontinent suffer similarly, growing rapidly fat on only modestly greater income.[18]

In the United States, as we will see in the next section, obesity is strongly correlated inversely with income. That is, poorer people are far more obese than wealthier ones. Historically, this pattern was not true in poorer countries, but it is becoming true. In South Africa, the population growing obese most quickly is poor Blacks.[19] In Brazil, where obesity is increasing rapidly, the most recent studies show that even as the obesity rate increased by 26 percent in women in the lower two income quintiles, it actually decreased by 10 percent in the higher quintiles.[20] As in wealthy countries, thinness is becoming a prominent marker of income and class.

The United States is just about the fattest country on Earth, but several of our Western counterparts are following closely. Canada, Germany, Australia, and the United Kingdom are close behind, although elderly people in the United Kingdom stay substantially slimmer than do elderly Americans.[21] In fact, it is easier to list wealthy nations that are actually staying *thin*. France, Italy, Japan, South Korea, and Norway are among the few countries with industrialized economies that are holding their obesity rates below 10 percent, and the rate in every one of these countries is rising, particularly among men.[22]

Susceptibility to an obesogenic environment is universal. A strong culture of traditional eating (France) and active living (Norway) can slow the march toward obesity, but ultimately, nearly everybody succumbs to the call of highly processed, over-sweetened foods and sedentary lives. Unless the environment is designed in such a way as to *prevent* people from indulging in gustatory excess, and to *force* people to move regularly, people will grow fat. We are simply too weak, or perhaps too human, to manage it on our own.

WEALTH AND CLASS DIFFERENCES

Wealth counts too, and it has for a long time. Although people who advocate for fat acceptance often emphasize that fat, historically, has been associated with wealth, the opposite has been true for some time in the

United States. As early as 1962, a research team led by Albert Stunkard at the University of Pennsylvania found that obesity was seven times as prevalent in women who had been raised in poor households than those raised in wealthy ones.[23] Moreover, obesity appeared to be dispositive for class mobility: 22 percent of downwardly mobile women were obese, versus 12 percent of upwardly mobile women.[24] And class-specific obesity started early, with only 7 percent of kindergarteners from the top-income quintile being obese, versus 17 percent from the bottom-income quintile. For girls, the differences were especially pronounced. By age six, obesity was nine times as prevalent in poor girls as wealthy girls.[25]

Obesity and class reinforce each other. Wealthier kids (and adults) are thinner, but thinner people (particularly women) tend to get wealthier. Thinner teenagers have a pronounced advantage in college admissions, job placement, and promotions. They network more successfully, accruing greater social capital through more powerful friends. Examples of workplace discrimination are legion, with fat women told over the phone that they are well qualified for a job, only to be turned down once they appear at the job site in person.[26] One study of students at selective colleges conducted in the late 1960s found them to be substantially thinner than the general pool of college-bound high school students. The fat kids had failed to make it through the admissions filter. "The only conclusion that we could arrive at," wrote the researchers, "was that marked discrimination is exercised by teachers and college interviewers against obese adolescents, especially females."[27] Jean Mayer, one of the study's two authors, later estimated that a fat boy had only one-half the chance of being admitted to a selective college as an academically comparable thin boy, while a fat girl had only one-third the chance.[28]

The reasons for the income gap in obesity are complex and elusive. Certainly, mental exhaustion and ego depletion play a role but so, too, do environment, peer effects, and social sanctions. Wealthier people are bathed in a culture of thinness where powerful social pressures threaten to ostracize individuals who exceed certain bodily proportions.[29] So intense is the pressure that wealthy, upper-middle-class *parents* admit to feeling morally judged on behalf of their overweight *children*. One nutrition writer wrote of the phenomenon: "Aerobicized, high-achieving adults don't want to display fat children. Fairly or not, parents are judged by their offspring, and these days, fat more than ever suggests sloth, improper eating habits, and a lack of education. . . . In a society where it seems that the poor eat potato chips and Big Macs while the better-off scarf down diet sodas and low-fat pretzels, obesity carries a powerful and unspoken message about social class."[30]

The poor tend to live immersed in bad-food environments, with fast-food restaurants being particularly accurate markers for low neighborhood incomes. Poor children are more likely to eat free or subsidized school lunches, which are often awful. When Ellen Haas, Assistant Secretary at the US Department of Agriculture under President Reagan, visited a school cafeteria in a poor urban neighborhood, she described the menu choices as, "french fries and pepperoni pizza . . . french fries and a steak and cheese sandwich . . . french fries and a fried-fish sandwich . . . and french fries and a submarine sandwich."[31]

Curiously, however, the environment seems to only have an impact on poor kids. Researchers who study the prevalence of obesity and proximity of fast-food restaurants find that the presence of more restaurants make children fatter, but only if the kids are poor. Rich kids seemed largely immune to their effect.[32] This is consistent with more general data showing that childhood obesity rates rose rapidly from 2001 to 2007, but only among kids from poor families. Again, the rich children seemed to be largely insulated from the effects of an obesogenic environment.[33] Similar

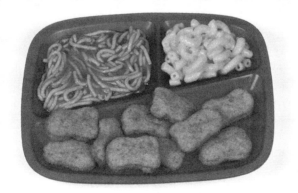

Lunches served in school cafeterias have been notoriously obesogenic. When a Reagan official visited several school cafeterias, she could find only french fries, fried fish, fried chicken, and pepperoni pizza. *Michael Neelon/Alamy Stock Photo*

effects were observed on army bases, where children of sergeants were fatter than children of commissioned officers (25 percent versus 15 percent), despite the fact that housing allowances and subsidized food made similar food choices economically feasible for all, regardless of income.[34]

The relationship between income (or class) and obesity is significant but not obvious. Rich kids and adults are much thinner than poor kids, and the disparity is getting starker in the twenty-first century. Poor kids live in more obesogenic environments to begin with, but they are also more vulnerable to toxic food environments than are rich kids. Whether through ignorance, peer pressure, lack of social consequences, or mental exhaustion brought by stress, poor kids are far less likely to resist fast-food restaurants and cheap fried food that suffuses their lives. Rich kids (and adults), subjected to intense peer pressure to remain thin, and more aware of the long-term costs of obesity in lost opportunities, networks, and romantic partners, are more successful at resisting the call. Moreover, as they resist the lure of bad food, and thus remain thinner, they open up opportunities to get richer still.

SOCIAL NETWORKS, FAMILIES, AND CLANS

Obesity tends to stick in groups, even in families. Children shun their obese classmates as playmates and look to each other for exercise cues.[35] Normal-weight teenagers show a pronounced preference to making friends with peers of similar weight, a phenomenon that sociologists call *homophily*.[36] Two researchers, Nicholas Christakis and James Fowler, have hypothesized that being friends with obese people leads to greater tolerance for the state of being obese and thus presages weight gain—a phenomenon that socially ambitious teenagers (particularly girls) know and avoid.[37] Mutual teenaged friends are twice as likely to grow obese if the other friend becomes obese, though in part this reflects a social distancing of people who are able to maintain their lower weights.[38] So powerful is the social effect that it largely trumps the impact of the physical environment. While it is true that nice weather, nearby parks, and exercise equipment help people to keep their weight down, these influences are easily overwhelmed by the presence of obese friends.[39]

Friends look to each other for cues on eating and exercise. The aerobics craze of the 1970s never really ended but, rather, morphed into Jazzercise, yoga, spinning, and running groups. People enjoy exercising together, and so choose friends who validate their exercise choices and goad each other to adhere to their regimens. Friends also seek out reinforcement on difficult eating choices—kale and tofu are simply more appealing when everybody around you is eating them too. As far back as 1953, a diet advice columnist recognized the phenomenon and encouraged his readers to seek friends to help them stick with their diets. He wrote, "A friend with the selfsame figure-control problem is a smarter choice than a slim-Jim who munches on anything edible, with no increase in waistline. Such provocation could end in homicide."[40]

Obesity runs in families, too. Fat spouses enable their spouses to be fat, or at least do not encourage them to be thin. In fact, marital discord can arise when a spouse loses a substantial amount of weight. "Fat is a family affair," wrote a researcher in 1975. "So is dieting."[41] In one disturbing study of fourteen couples where one spouse lost substantial amounts of weight following bariatric surgery, three couples divorced and the newly slim partner in several others had an extramarital affair. In three of the couples, the non-obese spouse strongly opposed the surgery, fearing that his or her partner would now have the latitude to roam. One newly thin wife admitted that her weight loss gave her the confidence to trade up to more high-functioning friends, to which her husband responded, "She's gotten it into her head that she's too good for anybody, and that includes me. . . . She probably is going to have an affair and go on and marry one of them."[42] Unexpectedly, sex, too, took a hit. Spouses felt insecure around their newly thin partners and feared that they were no longer adequate partners, sexually or otherwise. One man, describing his wife's newly revived libido, said, "We could use another man around the house to keep her rejuvenated."[43]

Obesity divides Americans in much the same way as do income and education, and the divides are self-reinforcing. Just as the well-educated and wealthy have become more adept at passing on their advantages to their children, ensuring that social benefits in the next generation will be distributed even more unequally, so do thin people now cement their social standing by bonding with other thin people and shunning the obese. Thin people support each other's good eating and exercise habits, and they cull the obese from their circles, depriving the obese of the exact sorts of role models and social support that they need to eat and exercise better. Coupled with geographical divides and ethnic and racial segregation, poor eating habits grow ever more firmly ensconced in socially disadvantaged groups who find it increasingly more difficult to make the profound changes in their lives that presage weight loss.

Overeating, like smoking and higher education, has become a power-ful class marker. The wealthy use their means to control their food environment so as to discourage obesity among themselves, their friends, and their children. Wealthy neighborhoods boast more gyms, more spin classes, fewer fast-food restaurants, and fewer donut shops. Trans fats were defeated at the barricades largely by highly educated and well-to-do mothers, just as teenage smoking and drunk driving were marginalized a generation ago. Powerful messages of ostracization or inclusion change the obesogenic environment and bend the weight curve. To quit drinking, almost everybody needs to stop hanging out in bars and avoid friends who drink. To lose weight, people need to avoid obesogenic loci and avoid friends who overeat and fail to exercise. Interestingly, challenging as it is to control a drinking habit, controlling an eating habit may be harder still.

11

What Is to Be Done?

WHAT HAVE WE LEARNED?

Readers who have gotten this far will wonder if there is anything to be done. While childhood obesity rates have recently stabilized, they are not declining. Over two-thirds of adults in the United States are overweight and obese. A conservative estimate puts the annual medical and disability cost of obesity in the United States at over $50 billion.[1] Our food environment tempts us with a near endless procession of cheap, high-sugar delights. Our built environment and life patterns are designed to funnel us from bed to easy chair to car to office chair to car to couch. As one alarmist gadfly wrote as early as 1974, "How do you get people to understand that millions of Americans have adopted diets that will make them at best fat, at worst dead?"[2]

One of the great challenges with responding to obesity is that the solution *appears* to be so simple: eat less and move more. The pure obviousness of the solution makes it difficult for us to take this epidemic seriously. However, a more rigorous analysis of the problem quickly disabuses us of its simplicity. The cost of obesity, for both the individual and society, is immense. Obesity dictates lower lifetime earnings, fewer professional opportunities, fewer promotions, fewer and worse marriage opportunities, diminished opportunities for education and training, fewer friends, extensive health problems, diminished pleasure, and diminished life expectancy. The cost to society in increased disability payments and health bills and in diminished productivity is also immense. The US Army, an outfit which has long had to confront the limits of America's youth in assembling a fighting force, views obesity as, quite literally, a threat to national security. If the solution were simple, we surely would have found it by now.

In understanding the limits of our potential response to the epidemic, I urge readers and policymakers to accept two unintuitive truths:

1. We have less control over what we eat and how we move than we think we do.

We have learned through both research and experience over the past several decades that when we change our food environment, we change how we eat. That is, our eating is largely a passive response to available food and not a volitional choice. While at any given moment we have the ability to exert control over what we consume, over long periods of time our eating habits adjust to the food around us. Our tastes, preferences, cravings, and habits are far more reactive than we tend to think. We eat what we are accustomed to eating, and we acclimate our eating habits to our environment. Thus, people who grow up in China prefer Chinese food, people who grow up in India prefer Indian food, and people who grow up in the American Midwest prefer Midwestern American food. We all start life with a fairly neutral palate, and then we habituate them to the food around us.

Our physical movements, too, are less volitional than we tend to think. In a preindustrial world, everybody walked, lifted, dug, wove, picked, hoed, weeded, threshed, ground, and mashed without thinking much of it. When life demanded that we dig for our supper, we all dug. When the calories were available to us without digging, we all stopped digging. Nobody digs for fun, and digging more than is necessary with the sole intent of simply burning off calories is, from an evolutionary standpoint, bizarre. We are programmed to conserve our calories, and we fall naturally to indolence when we are not impelled to move.

We can observe non-volitional movement in the ways people readily change their walking habits when they move to cities. People could walk around the parking lot of a suburban office park to intentionally burn off calories, but they don't. However, people naturally walk to work, or to the subway or bus stop, when such walking makes logistical sense. As we remove compelling reasons to move, most of us stop moving. The hundreds of micro-adjustments we have made to our environment to eliminate the necessity of moving—ranging from electric beaters to automatic car windows to television remote controls—have worked perfectly. Each advance has incrementally reduced the need to move, and we have responded each time by moving less. At this point, many of us hardly move at all. Daniel Lieberman, an evolutionary biologist who studies physical adaptation of the human body, notes that from a metabolic viewpoint, those of us who drive to sedentary office jobs never really get out of bed.[3]

If losing weight were simply a case of willpower, few of us would be fat. There is no evidence that we are less volitional or driven than we were a generation ago. However, if moving and eating are largely unconscious responses to the environment around us, then the more reasonable response must not be to change ourselves, but rather to change our environment. This leads me to the next point.

2. Our ability to resist temptation is limited.

Most of us, at one time or another, have forced ourselves to do hard things. We have held our tongues in a job interview, been on our best behavior on a first date, resisted sexual or gustatory temptation, and forced ourselves to cram for a test. Extraordinary challenges demand extraordinary responses, and most of us at some time in our lives have risen to the occasion.

We tend to recall those extraordinary efforts as proof that we are able to do hard things, and thus we blame ourselves for our inability to eat less and exercise more. However, the key word is "extraordinary." We evolved to be able to push ourselves, briefly, to overcome extremes. We did not evolve, however, to continually push ourselves to do hard things. Over time, we all fall back into preferred patterns.

Resisting tempting food is hard for most people, and doing it constantly is exhausting. The task is made all the more difficult when other components of our lives are also hard. We all have limited willpower to expend each day on resisting temptation and forcing ourselves to do difficult tasks. Those of us who enjoy sweet, high-fat foods (i.e., most of us) must expend high levels of psychic energy in our current food environment in not eating. This is simply unrealistic, particularly if work and family demands further deplete our mental reserves. To repeat Roy Baumeister's insight, willpower is "more than metaphor."

Likewise, forcing ourselves to move when there is no obvious need to do so is also ego depleting. Observations from the 1970s showed that the urge to move or not to is predetermined in most people. Dynamic people move naturally and without thinking about it. Sedentary people do not, and they must use limited powers of volition to force themselves to do so. (The reverse is also true. Office work is depleting for naturally restless people.) If you are a natural mover, you migrate intuitively to the stairs, to walking, and to active weekend pastimes. If you are not, each of these tasks requires you to deplete what limited willpower you have, leaving less resolve for the difficult chores of earning a living, battling with a bureaucracy, or raising children.

We are more responsive to our physical environment than we might think. All city people walk, even if they are naturally sluggish. They don't intentionally move to the suburbs in a purposeful effort to reduce the walking in their lives. However, once they find themselves in the suburbs, they intuitively mitigate their walking. It takes a highly purposeful person to resist the natural rhythms of her environment. We need to respond to this epidemic based on how people are, and not how they should be.

Adding impetus to this idea of non-volitional eating and moving is the recognition that bodyweight is more set than we might suppose. Multiple experiments on rats and observations of people show us that our bodies have a preferred level and distribution of fat, and that disrupting these set points requires inordinate effort. Observations of previously fat people who diet and maintain their weight loss show them to be physiologically starving. While they are not technically underweight, their bodies behave as though they are and reduce base metabolism rates accordingly.

Today we understand better how complex our satiation and hunger mechanisms are. Our neuroendocrine system has powerful tools at its disposal to force us to eschew food or crave it, and few people can long resist those cravings. Asking people to live productive lives while expending substantial willpower resisting food cravings in a food-rich environment is simply unrealistic. The answer must be to change the environment.

CHANGING OUR FOOD ENVIRONMENT

Changing our food environment requires profound changes in how we regulate food. At present, we regulate food only very lightly, demanding that the USDA set a floor for the freshness of highly perishable items such as meat and dairy products. We place few limits on the sale or consumption of unhealthy, quasi-addictive, or obesogenic foods, despite growing evidence that many of these foods more closely resemble narcotics than food. As I have discussed at length in earlier chapters, sugar is toxic in large doses over long periods of time. Kenneth Krause, a food scientist, writes that sugar "alters metabolism, raises blood pressure, causes hormonal chaos, and damages our livers. Like both tobacco and alcohol (a distillation of sugar) it affects our brains, encouraging us to increase consumption."[4]

Sugar is a dose-dependent toxin, and its effects accumulate over time. This is one reason why we have had such a hard time taking it seriously. People have been eating sugar for millennia, and in doses that are appropriate (and bound to fiber), it does us no harm. However, cheap, ubiquitous sugar today is playing havoc with our biology, our brain chemistry, our moods, and our weight-regulation systems. The answer must be not to outlaw the stuff but to regulate it reasonably. This means prohibiting sales of products with high levels of added sugars to children, regulating the size of packages and portions of certain products, limiting where specific products can be sold, and perhaps even placing warning signs on certain products. We would never, for example, allow whiskey to be sold in hardware stores, drug stores, and schools, and nor would we allow it to be sold in commercial sizes or to children. Yet we happily sell donuts, cookies, and candy in jumbo packages to children of all ages in every conceivable location. In fact, the Girl Scouts co-opt their charges to sell cookies door-to-door to raise money. The Boy Scouts could probably raise substantial funds selling cigarettes (or, in Colorado, marijuana) door-to-door, but we do not allow them to do it.

Regulating the sale of junk food might take the form of imposing high vice taxes on high-sugar products to dissuade price-sensitive children from buying them, or moving certain products behind the counter and demanding that IDs be shown to buy them. Or perhaps it might mean limiting the sizes that products can be sold in. No ten-year-old ought to be allowed to buy a pound of red licorice, just as we do not allow adults to buy a twenty-four-ounce martini.

We might experiment with other sorts of regulations as well. For example, we can require that portion sizes be consistent to help consumers compare costs and calories over different locales and to undercut the tendency of restaurants to "super-size" in an effort to build loyalty.[5] We can outlaw all-you-can-eat buffets and refillable sodas, ban foods from certain public areas, or limit food and drink to certain times of the day. We can certainly ban food from certain obvious public places like subways, buses, trains, theaters, parks, and schools, except in specifically delineated dining cars, picnic areas, and lunchrooms. Although all of this sounds quite radical, we have only recently allowed food and drink into many of these areas.

Changing our food environment means changing our food habits as well. As a society, we need to revert to older eating patterns: at designated times and places, usually with other people. While we cannot require that people eat together, we can take action to facilitate healthier eating habits like incorporating cooking classes into schools for all students, banning school activities during a two-hour dinner period, and expanding lunch periods. Eating on-the-run, a toxic practice, can be undermined through prohibiting eating in many public areas where people currently do so. In short, while we do not want to ban certain eating habits, we need to make many of the least healthy eating habits harder, less convenient, more circumscribed, and more expensive. I would not want to live in a society where I cannot occasionally indulge in a hot fudge sundae, nor do I wish to live in one where donuts and candy bars beckon to me constantly and where no place in my day is food-free. The idea is not so much to ban the donuts as, in the words of Deborah Cohen, "to put the donuts a little further out of reach."[6]

CHANGING OUR PHYSICAL ENVIRONMENT

Moving cannot be conditional on getting people to the gym. Most people hate the gym, and a weekend softball game or a round of golf is hardly adequate to significantly raise the amount of energy that people expend. Rather, the solution for many people must come from integrating walking into their days, and this will require not just changing the built environment but the entire rhythm of the day.

Americans love suburbia, so the answer cannot be to have 100 million Americans move into walk-up flats in the city. Rather, the solution must be to modify suburbs as to make them more centralized and walkable: more similar to the original railroad suburbs of a century ago. This movement is already taking off, with many suburban towns redesigning their cores to be more pedestrian-friendly and designed around the principals of new-urbanism. Towns can build denser housing around bus and rail stations, create new zoning to allow mixed-use residential and commercial space and relocate parking behind stores so as to create more walkable retail districts. Historically, this was the way we built our suburbs, and there is evidence that many Americans would welcome a return to more a communal and walkable living environment if they could preserve the quiet and privacy that comes from suburban living. The two are not mutually exclusive. Private space can coexist with a public sphere, and by many accounts, Americans would like a happier marriage of the two.

Some of this will only happen slowly, as existing housing decays and opportunities arise to rethink and redesign our towns. However, part of this can be done on a more accelerated schedule. Public transportation is consistently starved for the sake of our automobile infrastructure, and archaic zoning regulations continue to bar planners from putting housing above retail spaces, schools and churches next to homes, and stores and homes abutting streets rather than buffered by parking lots and ornamental lawns. Zoning can be changed, infrastructure redeveloped, and rail lines improved. Cities in South America and Europe have developed exclusive lanes for commuter busses, prepay stations to move busses through streets more quickly, high-speed commuter rails, and sophisticated car and bike-sharing arrangements. Anything that moves people out of private cars tends to promote walking, and the cycle is self-reinforcing. As more people walk, they create a greater market for pedestrian-designed infrastructure and retail. And as fewer people drive, bus transportation becomes more efficient.

Lastly, gas and parking taxes can also push people to public transportation, just as vice taxes can dissuade people from indulging. The great gift to New York City's public transportation system is the sky-high cost of parking in Manhattan. Only the wealthiest commuters can afford parking, which can approach $1,000 per month in midtown. Parking tends to be private, and prices float to the market, but gas is heavily taxed in most places in the world, pushing people to drive less, to carpool, and to utilize smaller cars when they do drive. Americans have gotten used to heavily subsidized private driving (with our free highways and cheap municipal lots) and have responded rationally: by driving. Different policies and taxes can induce different behavior, with the multiple benefits of lowering exhaust and carbon emissions while improving health.

CHANGING OUR LIFE HABITS

Eating thin means living thin; this requires changes more profound than simply taking smaller portions and eschewing dessert. Our eating habits flow from our daily life patterns. We need to teach our kids to eat differently from a young age, which entails introducing more complex flavors and food textures to them repeatedly while refusing to placate them with sweet and simple carbohydrates. Such food education is costly in time and effort and requires a greater societal commitment to steady and consistent mealtime standards. The endless stream of pizza and cupcake parties that have become part of the American childhood experience do more than make children fat; they undermine our efforts to expand our children's palates.

Americans avoid exercise and cooking through ignorance, but also because they are exhausted, stressed, and strapped for time. Exercise, cooking, walking, and preparing and consuming group meals all take time, and this time has to be carved from other daily activities. While American children can spend less time watching screens, the adults need to steal time from commuting or working, which requires more profound change. People consider many factors for structuring their lives, but one thing they rarely think about is the extra pounds that they and their children will put on if they are spending extra hours each day commuting. Americans study property tax bills and school rankings carefully when choosing a home; perhaps it would be helpful to place an obesity statistic on a house listing that will show how much weight you can expect you and your children to gain if extra hours are lost to commuting.

A similar calculus holds for extra work hours. Overworked adults speak of the time robbed from their friends and family by the extra hours they work, but they tend to ignore the hours taken from exercise and food preparation. As many Americans are in daily energy imbalance of about 150 calories, they need to integrate one and a half additional miles of walking into their day, which takes about thirty minutes for most adults. That thirty minutes can come out of work, commuting, socializing, or screen time, but it must come out of somewhere. If family and work obligations are inflexible, then a longer commute may be the deciding factor.

The same holds for children. Amish children, the thinnest of all American children, participate in almost no organized sports. They do, however, walk nearly everywhere and thus burn off more than enough calories to offset their food intake. For many of our children, poorly designed physical education classes in schools are simply inadequate to compensate for their excess daily calories.[7] Moreover, the much-celebrated varsity athletics in American high schools, which do provide vigorous workouts for children, are accessible to only a very small portion of students.

Few of our children walk or bike to school. Rain and snow have come to be seen as non-negotiable barriers for children. Safety and liability standards now dissuade parents from allowing their children to walk on moderately busy streets or during even perfectly safe hours during daylight. Schools rarely promote walking and bicycling or even make allowances by installing bicycle racks. Moreover, schools are rarely situated in deliberately walkable neighborhoods, where large numbers of children can get to school on their own.

Getting thin will require examining every component of our lives to facilitate eating and moving differently. Given the tremendously high rate of obese and overweight individuals in the United States today, we ought to start with the assumption that almost nothing we are doing today is working. Our living and work choices, family dynamics, and perceptions about optimizing time for both ourselves and our children have led to catastrophic obesity rates while nearly guaranteeing shorter lives for the next generation. Almost all aspects of our days ought to be up for scrutiny and potential change. Simply eating more carrots is a woefully inadequate response.

WHAT DOESN'T WORK

Some misconceptions about obesity make fighting it all that much harder. Certain types of physical activities and approaches to physical education do little good and sometimes lead to harm. Healthier food choices may be better for your heart without cutting calories from your diet. Various approaches to nutrition education seem to produce little benefit, and certain methods that have been long dismissed as potentially harmful, like overt social pressure, may be more useful than we wish to admit. Public service advertising accomplishes almost nothing.

Perhaps no idea has been as pervasive, or as unhelpful, as the "food desert"—those urban poverty zones with no supermarkets and few places to buy fresh produce. The food desert explanation appeals to classic anti-poverty advocates because it suggests that the key to obesity is simply purchasing power: If we could simply get enough cash into the hands of poor people, they could buy better food and thereby get thinner. However, obesity is more an artifact of what we *do* eat than what we *don't*. It is more important to eat fewer candy bars and refined starchy foods and to drink less fruit juice than it is to eat more fruits and vegetables. While it is true fructose bound to fiber is better than unbound fructose (i.e., white sugar), what would be better is to not eat fructose at all. (No mangos are better than one mango.) Similarly, if vegetables displace starches and sugars, then they are a welcome addition to the diet; but if vegetables are simply added to a starch-laden diet, they will do little beyond possibly controlling spiking insulin levels.

Americans, with their consumerist culture, seem obsessed with the idea of finding the right food to buy and consume, but the better response is to simply consume less. Better food produces slimness when it displaces worse food, and thus leads to greater satiation with fewer calories. However, too many poverty advocates push vegetables as a complement to a starchy diet. The few studies done of making better produce available in poor neighborhoods have shown little to no effect from the effort.

We saw this phenomenon in the 1980s with the movement toward low-fat foods (which simply substituted in high-sugar foods), and we saw it again in the concerted efforts in the last decade to remove trans fats from processed foods. Trans fats attracted an extraordinary level of media scrutiny given their toxic effects on levels of low-density lipoproteins (LDLs, aka the "bad" cholesterol), yet substituting healthier cis fats for trans fats did nothing to alleviate obesity. This was a matter of people believing that eating the *right* thing was better than eating nothing, which in the case of obesity (and its attendant diabetes) is almost never true.[8]

The varsity athlete, with which America has almost an obsessive fascination, produces almost no benefit in combatting obesity. Varsity sports programs tend to select a small group of promising athletes at young ages (traveling teams are starting as young as eight years old in some suburban leagues) and invest inordinate resources in training these young athletes, largely at the expense of investing in more accessible sports programs aimed at non-elite athletic children. In fact, insofar as they command athletic budgets and encourage most children to become spectators rather than players, varsity programs actually hurt physical fitness in the young. Justifications for varsity sports programs rarely emphasize the spillover athletic effect on to a student body. Rather, the claimed benefits usually include increased morale and enhanced school pride and spirit.[9]

This is not an argument against team sports but rather an argument against undue emphasis placed on team sports at the expense of more inclusive sporting programs for non-elite athletes. Recreation programs, hiking and running clubs, swim teams, tennis and rowing programs, and various youth leagues in team sports such as softball, baseball, basketball, volleyball, and soccer can teach many more children the pleasures of competition and athleticism and produce in them lifetime habits of fitness. The key here, as is true with almost everything having to do with obesity, is sustainability. The goal is to get kids accustomed to strenuously using their bodies and enjoying the experience. Certain sports, tackle football, in particular, are rarely sustained into adulthood and almost never played in an unorganized program, and thus they are poor candidates for producing lifelong habits of fitness.

Anti-junk food advertising, and indeed food education in general, produces little effect in combatting obesity. This harkens back to the material that I presented in earlier chapters showing that much of our eating is unconscious and that almost all of it responds to the environment. Food education as a tactic in combating obesity presupposes that people eat thoughtfully, yet almost everything we know about eating suggests that the opposite is the case. People eat in response to available food choices, containers, plates, portion sizes, social cues, environmental cues, stress, smells, tactile stimuli, and time of day. They rarely eat in response to their own hunger, much less in compliance with objective nutrition information. Posting calories in restaurants seems to have no effect on food choice. In fact, one dispiriting study showed that people ate *more* calories after restaurants started posting calorie counts next to menu items.

Education does help but not nutrition education. Rather, the most effective education is more akin to behavioral therapy: training people to contort their personal surroundings into less obesogenic environments. This involves eating at home more, using smaller plates, leaving serving dishes on the counter (rather than at the table), eating with friends, avoiding processed foods, turning off the television during meals, and eating foods with more complex flavors. That is, as eating thinner necessitates living thinner, we need to learn how to live thinner rather than learn more about the nutrition content of food.

Lastly, one solution to obesity has been to simply ignore it. "Fat acceptance" advocates have emerged periodically to argue that fat is not the problem but rather that our attitude toward fat is. In one of my favorite examples of this genre, Margaret Deirdre O'Hartigan wrote in 1994:

> Call me a bodybuilder, for lack of a better term. Bodybuilders treat their bodies as living sculpture, a plastic medium to develop to the fullest their idea of physical perfection. That's what I can do: I deliberately overeat to give my body the plushest, most voluptuous contours I can acquire.

Growing fatter is one of the most intensely sensuous things that I have ever
experienced. I love the sensation of eating beyond satiation almost as much
as I love the subsequent expansion of my entire body. The fatter I grow, the
more exquisitely attuned to my own body and to the feel of another's touch
I become. There is no small amount of satisfaction for me in seeing a lover's
eyes widen in amazement at my growing bulk. But growing fatter is first and
foremost a matter of loving myself, and only secondarily a form of erotic
expression that I want to share with my lover.[10]

While this book is certainly not an argument against sensuality of any
sort, fat acceptance movements ignore the objective evidence that obesity
kills and that one of the tools that societies use to fight obesity is to help
their members to cleave to conforming norms surrounding eating. I do
not mean that society should demonize overweight people, but rather that
society should encourage all of its members to strive to maintain a healthy
weight. People striving to change their lives and eating habits need love
and support, and they need acceptance of their worth as individuals. However, validating the worth of the individual is not tantamount to validating
all of their choices and behaviors.

WE'VE BEEN HERE BEFORE . . .

If my ideas seem like an overreach of a nanny-state government, I must
point out that we are closely paralleling efforts of fifty years ago to regulate tobacco. Tobacco, like sugar, was and is a legal and natural product.
Like sugar, it was available virtually everywhere to anybody who cared to
buy it. Like sugar, it was largely unregulated. People of all ages could buy
cigarettes, and people could smoke cigarettes in almost all places at all
times. People smoked at home and in the office, in parks and restaurants,
on planes, trains, and busses, and in hospitals and nursing homes. So pervasive was tobacco that most non-smokers kept ashtrays in their homes so
as to be able to more graciously attend to their guests who smoked.

Although Americans had smoked since the first European settlers encountered tobacco, the practice did not become widespread until after
World War I when returning servicemen, inducted into the habit through
cheap army-issued cigarettes, brought their new habit back to civilian life.
Smoking rates rose sharply among men over the following four decades
and among women after World War II. From the 1920s to the 1960s, consumption of cigarettes in the United States rose from 750 per adult per year

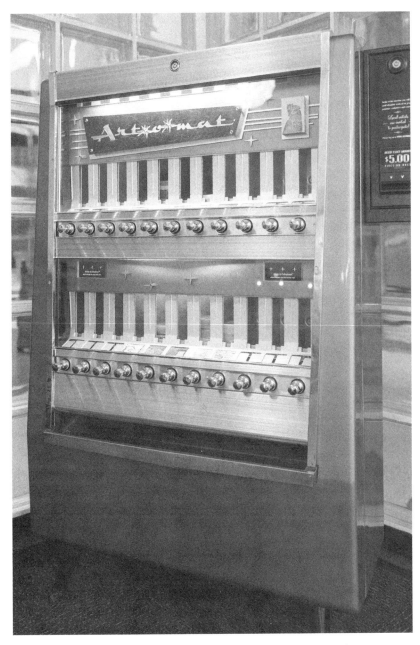

Little more than a generation ago, cigarettes were sold in vending machines most everywhere. Although the law forbade sale to minors, few states enforced the injunction. *Philip Scalia/Alamy Stock Photo*

to 3,900. By the 1960s, nearly 50 percent of adult Americans smoked; the oldest had been smoking at that point for forty-five years.

Hard as it is to believe, most Americans thought the habit to be safe. There is a good reason for this, as tobacco tends to produce its most toxic effects only after decades of smoking. In 1920, for example, the rate of lung cancer in the United States was just two per 100,000 adults, and by 1935, it had only risen to six per 100,000 despite the sharp rise in smoking beginning in 1916. However, by 1954, the rate had risen to twenty-three per 100,000: a twelvefold increase in the natural prevalence in the population. Forty years of smoking was producing its inevitable consequence.[11]

From early on, a few insightful health watchers suspected that smoking was toxic. A French physician reported in 1859 that of the sixty-eight cancer patients in his local hospital (mostly of the oral cavity), sixty-six smoked pipes, and one chewed tobacco. In 1936, two physicians in New Orleans, Alton Ochsner and Michael DeBakey, observed that nearly all of their lung cancer patients were smokers, and two years later, Raymond Pearl of Johns Hopkins noted that his patients who smoked tended to die younger. In 1939, Ángel Roffo of Argentina reported that he had produced cancer in rabbits by painting cigarette extracts on their bare skin.[12]

By the late 1950s, many physicians had given up smoking, even if their patients had not. On a daily basis, they observed rising rates of lung cancer, heart disease, and emphysema and associated the rising incidence of these diseases with smoking. Many physicians found pre-cancerous lesions and growths on the tongues and gums of many of their patients who were long-time smokers. In that same decade, physicians observed that smoking "accelerates the heart rate, raises the blood pressure, increases the work of the heart, and constricts the blood vessels of the extremities."[13] The American Cancer Society reported that in a study of 187,000 men between the ages of fifty and seventy, heavy smokers died from coronary heart disease twice as frequently as men who had never smoked, and they concluded that cigarette smoking was, ". . . an important, or even the major, factor contributing to the development of lung cancer."[14] "The most important finding of this study," wrote the authors, "was the high degree of association between cigarette smoking and the total death rate."[15]

What is important to recognize is that by the late 1950s, or the early 1960s at the latest, a small core of scientifically informed people understood that smoking was lethal, even as most of the population failed to recognize the fact. In the early 1960s, E. Cuyler Hammond, the principal author of the American Cancer Society study, had pathologists examine hundreds of slides of lung tissue from both smokers and non-smokers. To a near perfect degree, the pathologists were able to identify which samples had come from people who had smoked, and they could even reliably estimate how heavily the people had smoked.[16] Doctors who were able to began giving up smoking, and almost all acknowledged the dangers inherent in the habit. By 1964, when United States Surgeon General Luther Terry released his famous *Smoking and Health: Report of the Advisory Committee to the Surgeon General of the United States*, almost all medically trained people were already aware of the data.[17]

Similarly with the processed-food industry today, one response of the tobacco industry was to try to make their products safer, first by adding filters to cigarettes and later by marketing "low-tar" and "low-nicotine" formulations. Lorillard introduced Kent filter-tip cigarettes with an aggressive advertising campaign suggesting that the filter removed cancerous elements from the smoke. Competing firms followed with their own filter-tipped cigarettes. Liggett & Myers advertised their new L&Ms, "No filter compares with L&M's pure white Miracle Tip . . . *much more* flavor, *much less* nicotine."[18]

The parallels with today are striking. Just as removing all of the fat from food makes it unappealing, removing the tar and nicotine from cigarette smoke made smoking about as appealing as "a puff of warm air," in the words of one skeptic.[19] Moreover, just as processed food manufacturers compensated for the lost fat by adding extra sugar, thus negating any health effect of the lower-fat formulations, cigarette manufacturers counterbalanced the filtering effects by increasing the levels of nicotine in their cigarettes. More importantly, the filters seemed to reassure nervous smokers that their vice was not harmful and that they could thus ignore warnings with impunity. By 1963, even as large numbers of the most informed strata of citizens were turning away from tobacco, levels of smoking reached a new high. Tobacco companies sold 530 billion cigarettes that year.[20]

An infusion of corporate money misled the public and delayed smoking cessation for millions. In the early 1960s, the tobacco industry grossed $8 billion annually, spent $150 million on advertising, and contributed $3 billion in taxes to federal and state treasuries.[21] Amazingly, even as the Surgeon General's report warned Americans away from tobacco, tobacco growers were receiving $40 million annually in federal subsidies as a "protected crop." Thus industry, state treasurers, tobacco growers, and even federal agencies all had a vested interest in preserving Americans' existing smoking habits. The same was true in other countries. Tobacco taxes in the

United Kingdom, for example, contributed 822 million pounds sterling, just about half of that country's annual defense expenditure.[22] Tobacco companies responded to the scare posed by the Surgeon General's report by increasing their advertising budgets to $200 million annually, much of it aimed at adolescents who were most susceptible to the wiles of advertising and most vulnerable to the lure of smoking. Using such slogans as, "Luckies separate the men from the boys," ad agencies managed to raise smoking still farther.[23] Even a nationwide 1970 ban on television advertising of tobacco products could not slow the advertising juggernaut; the industry simply responded by increasing their advertising in print, on busses, and on billboards fivefold. By 1972, the outdoor advertising budget alone was greater than the budget for all print outlets had been before the television ban. Cigarette smoking, incredibly, actually increased in the years after the ban to $585 billion per year, a "testimony to the habituating capacity of cigarettes, and to the merchandizing skill of the cigarette manufacturing and marketing industry," in the words of one industry observer.[24]

However, the message finally was out. Cigarette smoking declined precipitously in the following decades. Rates of smoking by teenagers declined sharply in the 1980s, followed by declining adult smoking a decade later. Local ordinances made cigarette smoking progressively more costly and less convenient. In many states and cities, smoking was banned in restaurants, parks, workplaces, and government buildings. Smoking was banned on rail travel and domestic flights of two hours or less (and later on international flights as well). Almost all retailers who sold cigarettes began to require proof of age to purchase them; cigarette vending machines were outlawed nationwide.

Today, only about 15 percent of American adults smoke, which is down from 43 percent in 1965. Smoking is disallowed in almost all public places; New York City has even banned it from bars. Rates continue to decline at about 1 percent a year.

The nation's lengthy change in smoking habits, and in its attitude toward regulating tobacco sales and use, provide for us a template for progress on obesity. As was true in the early 1960s for tobacco, a small group of scientifically and medically informed Americans is aware of the dangers of our current food environment and our present eating habits, even while most Americans continue to ignore warning signs, such as the rising rates of diabetes and heart disease. As was true in the mid-1960s, the processed-food industry is using its advertising muscle to misinform the public about

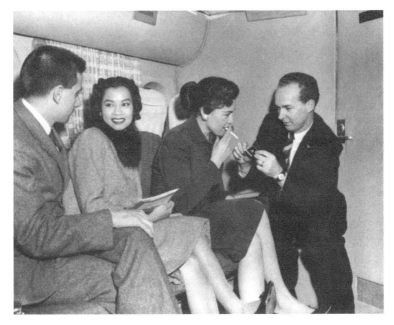

Smoking on commercial airplanes was allowed until a generation ago. It was banned on domestic flights of less than two hours in 1988 and on all flights over the following decade. *Getty Images*

the dangers of continuing with our present consumption of sugar and processed food, and they are pressuring government agencies to ignore the threats of overeating. And as in the 1960s, libertarian-minded Americans are offended at the idea that the state should play a role in regulating a dangerous behavior that many people think of as a "personal choice."

The landscape is slowly beginning to change. A recent poll of Americans in seventy-five counties from around the country found that 68 percent approve of increased government regulation of sugared beverages in an effort to combat obesity.[25] Public school systems in wealthier school districts are banning the sale of sugar-sweetened beverages and candy bars in cafeteria vending machines. Various activist parent groups have lobbied to halt bake sales as fundraising events and, similarly, to turn away from candy and cookie sales.[26] The nation's attitude toward regulating toxic food is paralleling its attitude toward regulating tobacco from fifty years ago, with the most progressive-minded and scientifically informed Americans most receptive to government action. Continued education and social adaptation may lead to further acceptance of regulation and perhaps, ultimately, to outright bans or heavy taxes on certain forms of sugar and processed food, such as "bottomless" and jumbo-sized soft drinks, jumbo candy packages, and unregulated sales of cookies and candy to minors. We may come, too, to print health warnings on many food and restaurant products and to hold vendors liable for health effects suffered by consumers.

Fighting the obesity epidemic will require a radical change in our attitude toward food and eating. We will need to view many types of food as potentially dangerous, requiring caution and regulation. We will need to think much more strategically about such life choices as our employment, housing, family structure, habits of daily living, locomotion, commuting, and recreational activities. There may come a time when we respond with horror to stories of friends spending the day on a couch watching television, just as we today look back in shock at nineteenth-century tales of multi-day binges in a local opium den. We will need to reconsider our education systems, our embracing of choice, and the limits of parental authority over children's eating habits. We will need to redesign our built environments and reconsider our perceptions of appropriate automobile use. We will need to rethink the costs of tolerating overly long work shifts, over-scheduled children, and disrupted family mealtimes. That is, we will need to do all of this if we wish to lose weight and prevent our children from dying prematurely.

If we continue on our current trajectory, we have every reason to believe that our present problem will grow worse. Given our natural inclination to sloth, our rapacious appetite for sugar and simple starches, our hyper-mechanized and unwalkable environments, our sedentary work styles, and our inadequate control over our own eating, there is little to stop us from growing ever fatter. Diabetes, heart disease, joint pain, physical discomfort, professional and social failure, and early death await us if we continue as we have been.

Notes

CHAPTER 1

1. "Obesity is Now No. 1 U.S. Nutritional Problem," *Science News Letter*, 12/27/52, p. 408.

2. From L. L. Williams, *Obesity*, Oxford University Press, 1926, as quoted in David Barr, "Health and Obesity," *NEJM*, 248:23, 6/4/53, p. 967.

3. David Barr, "Health and Obesity," *NEJM*, 248:23, 6/4/53, p. 967.

4. "Fat and Unhappy," *Time*, 50:16, 10/20/47.

5. Howard Rusk, "Overweight: Our Primary Health Problem," *NYT*, 11/30/52.

6. "Fat and Unhappy," *Time*, 59:25, 6/23/52.

7. Reported in "Diabetes Up?", *Time*, 50:14, 10/6/47.

8. Quoted in Thomas Desmod, "Fat Men Can't Win," *Science Illustrated*, June 1949, p. 46.

9. John Kelly, "Are We Becoming a Nation of Weaklings?" *American Magazine*, vol. 161, March, 1956, p. 28.

10. Thomas Merimee, "Obesity and Hyperinsulinism," *NEJM*, 285:15, 10/7/71, p. 856.

11. Lloyd Kolbe of the University of Texas, quoted in John Carey and Mary Hager, "Failing in Fitness," *Newsweek*, 4/1/85, p. 84.

12. *Ibid.*

13. Tina Alder, "US Adults: A Weighty Lot," *Science News*, vol. 146, 7/23/94, p. 53.

14. Quoted in Anastasia Toufexis, "Dieting: The Losing Game," *Time*, vol. 127, 1/20/86.

15. Smaller countries, such as some in Polynesia, may have been fatter but reliable statistics were elusive.

16. Cited in Philip Abelson and Donald Kennedy, "The Obesity Epidemic," *Science*, vol. 304, 6/4/04. There was some evidence, though hardly conclusive evidence, that rates of obesity were plateauing by 2010. See Susan and Jack Yanovski, "Obesity Prevalence in the United States: Up, Down, or Sideways," *NEJM*, vol. 364, 3/17/11, p. 987.

17. Wayne Millar and Thomas Stephens, "The Prevalence of Overweight and Obesity in Britain, Canada, and the United States," *AJPH*, 77:1, January 1987, p. 38–41.

18. Ali Mokdad, Mary Serdula, et al., "The Spread of the Obesity Epidemic in the United States, 1991–1998," *JAMA*, 282:16, 10/27/99, p. 1519–22.

19. Gina Kolata, "Obese Children: A Growing Problem," *Science*, vol. 232, 4/4/86, p. 20–21. Also, Solveig Cunningham, Michael Kramer, and K. M. Venkat Narayan, "Incidence of Childhood Obesity in the United States," *NEJM*, vol. 370, 1/30/14, p. 403–11.

20. *Ibid.*

21. Quoted in Jerry Adler and Claudia Kalb "An American Epidemic: Diabetes," *Newsweek*, 136:10, 9/4/00, p. 40–47.

22. Quoted in David Kessler, *The End of Overeating*, Rodale, 2009, p. 171.

23. David Ludwig, "Childhood Obesity—The Shape of Things to Come," *NEJM*, vol. 357, 12/6/07, p. 2325–27.

24. John Sullivan, "What is Obesity?" *Science Digest*, June 1985.

25. Chapter 2 describes type II diabetes in greater detail, but the reader should be aware that knowledge of an essential mechanism in type II is missing: How does obesity negate the catalytic effect of insulin? There are numerous theories, but no one has been proven conclusively.

26. Today we would call it "fatty liver syndrome." See Herbert Schreier, "Obesity," *Hygeia*, February 1946.

27. A. Master, L. Dublin, and H. Marks, "Normal Blood Pressure Range and its Clinical Implications," *JAMA*, 143:17, 1950, p. 1464–70. See also, L. Dublin, D. Armstrong, G. Wheatley, and H. Marks, "Obesity and its Relation to Health and Disease," *JAMA*, 147:11, 1951, p. 1007–14.

28. Quoted in Miriam Zeller Gross, "Why Fat People Die Sooner," *Hygeia*, February, 1949. See also, Louis Dublin, "Overweight: America's Number 1 Health Problem," *Today's Health*, September 1952.

29. Ingrid Nelson, "What is Obesity?" *Science Digest*, June 1985, p. 28.

30. Robert Lustig, *Fat Chance*, Plume, 2012, p. 5. See also, David Allison, Raffaella Zannolli, and K. M. Venkat Narayan, "The Direct Health Care Costs of Obesity in the United States," *AJPH*, 89:8, August 1999, p. 1194–99. The one mitigating factor was that obese people tended to die younger, and thus drew fewer Social Security and Medicare benefits over their lifetimes.

31. Eliot Marshall, "Public Enemy Number One: Tobacco or Obesity," *Science*, 304:5672, 5/7/04, p. 804.

32. Connie Colabro, "I Hated My Looks Until I Lost Forty Pounds," *Ladies Home Journal*, vol. 73, August 1956, p. 56.

33. Gina Kolata, "Obese Children: A Growing Problem," *Science*, vol. 222, 4/4/86.

34. Elizabeth Hurlock, "Psychological Problems of Overweight," *Today's Health*, April 1957, p. 62.

35. Cited in Lustig, *Fat Chance*, p. 23.

36. Quoted in Ellen Buzbee, "Future in the Scale," *NYT Magazine*, 3/12/67, p. 283.

37. The researchers controlled for test scores and high school grades. Helen Canning and Jean Mayer, "Obesity—Its Possible Effect on College Acceptance," *NEJM*, 275:21, 11/24/66; also, "Discrimination: Weighty Problem," *Newsweek*, 3/31/75, p. 64.

38. Quoted in Anastasia Toufexis, "Dieting: The Losing Game," *Time*, vol. 127, 1/20/86, p. 54. See, also, Krista Casaza, Kevin Fontaine, et al., "Myths Presumptions, and Facts about Obesity," *NEJM*, vol. 368, 2/5/13, p. 446–54.

39. Thomas Desmond, "Fat Men Can't Win," *Science Illustrated*, June 1949, p. 47.

40. Quoted in Anastasia Toufexis, "The Shape of the Nation," *Time*, vol. 126, 10/7/85, p. 60.

41. See Gina Kolata, "Death Rates Rising for Middle-Aged White Americans," *NYT*, 11/2/15. The rising death rate was due to a number of factors, including drug use, alcoholism, and suicide, in addition to heart disease.

CHAPTER 2

1. Readers interested in the evolutionary development of the human body may wish to consult Daniel Lieberman, *The Story of the Human Body*, Pantheon, 2013, particularly Chapter 10. See also Michael Power and Jay Schulkin, *The Evolution of Obesity*, Johns Hopkins Press, 2009.

2. Vincent Dole, "Body Fat," *Scientific American*, December 1959, vol. 201, p. 42.

3. Power and Schulkin, p. 62.

4. "Why Fat People Die Sooner," *Hygeia*, 27:2, February 1949.

5. S. Boyd Easton, Marjorie Shostak, and Melvin Konner, *The Paleolithic Prescription*, Harper and Row, 1988.

6. One interesting case study is of the !Kung tribe of the Kalahari Desert. Nomadic until the 1960s, tribesmen had minimal inflammatory or heart disease and virtually no obesity or diabetes. A rapid transition to agriculturalism has led to increased obesity, joint and heart disease, and age-related high blood pressure. See Gina Kolata, "!King Hunter-Gatherers: Feminism, Diet, and Birth Control," *Science*, vol. 185, 9/13/74, p. 932–34.

7. Jessica Selinger of Simon Fraser University has found that people subconsciously adjust their motions and strides so as to conserve energy. See Jessica Selinger, Shawn O'Connor, et al., "Humans Can Continuously Optimize Energetic Cost During Walking," *Current Biology*, 25:18, 9/21/15, p. 2452–56.

8. Ryan Jaslow, "80 Percent of American Adults Don't Get Recommended Exercise," CBS News, May 3, 2013, http://www.cbsnews.com/news/cdc-80 -percent-of-american-adults-dont-get-recommended-exercise/.

9. Joan Bulfer and C. Eugene Allen, "Fat Cells and Obesity," *BioScience*, 29:12, 12/79, p. 736–41.

10. Susan Ozanne, "Epigenetic Signatures of Obesity," *NEJM*, 372:10, 3/5/15, p. 973–74.

11. "Why Kids Stay Fat," *Newsweek*, 10/19/70, p. 83.

12. Joanne Silberner, "Baby Fat," *Science News*, vol. 131, 1/31/87.

13. Gina Kolata, "Why Do People Get Fat?" *Science*, 227:4692, 3/15/85, p. 1327–28.

14. Met Life researchers found a 20 percent decline in mortality among men who lost even a modest amount of weight, relative to their counterparts who stayed at the same weight. See Louis Dublin, "Overweight: America's No. 1 Health Problem," *Today's Health*, November 1952.

15. Richard Ostlund, Myrlene Staten, et al., "The Ratio of Waist-to-Hip Circumference Plasma Insulin Level, and Glucose Intolerance as Independent Predictors of the HDL2 Cholesterol Level in Older Adults," *NEJM*, 322:4, 1/25/90, p. 229–34.

16. Ingrid Wickelgren, "Do 'Apples" Fare Worse Than 'Pears'?" *Science*, 280:5368, 5/29/98, p. 1365.

17. "Why Fat People Die Sooner," *Hygeia*, February 1949. It's difficult to know precisely when the first researcher connected abdominal fat with heart disease. French researcher Jean Vauge postulated the relationship in 1947, but Met Life actuaries had already observed the statistical correlation.

18. Described in David Freedman, "Obesity: Waist Not, But Okay Behind," *Science News*, vol. 137, 5/26/90.

19. Reported in Joanne Silberner, "Fat Distribution and Heart Disease," *Science News*, vol. 127, 1/26/85.

20. John Elliot, "Blame It All on Brown Fat Now," *JAMA*, 243:20, 5/23/80, p. 1983–85.

21. Nancy Rothwell and Michael Stock, "A Role for Brown Adipose Tissue in Diet-Induced Thermogenesis," *Nature*, vol. 281, September 6, 1979, p. 31–35.

22. Sidney Abraham and Marie Nordsieck, "Relationship of Excess Weight in Children and Adults," *PHR*, 75:3, March 1960, p. 263–73.

23. Gail Fisher and Helen Vavra, "Screening High-Yield Groups for Diabetes," *PHR*, 80:11, November 1965, p. 961–68.

24. See, for example, Ilonna and Alfred Rimm, "Association Between Juvenile Onset Obesity and Severe Adult Obesity in 73,532 Women," *AJPH*, 66:5, May, 1976.

25. Quoted in Diane Edwards, "Body Shape: In the Eye of the Receptor?" *Science News*, vol. 133, 1/23/88, p. 54. It's worth noting that slim youths can turn fat—particularly women post-pregnancy. One study of overweight women in their 50s found that just over a third had not been overweight up until age 20. Either pregnancy permanently re-sets certain sorts of feedback mechanisms or (more likely) raising children fulltime tends to drive many women to eat more than they otherwise would. See Arthur Hartz and Alfred Rimm, "Natural History of Obesity in 6,946 Women Between 50 and 59 Years of Age," *AJPH*, 70:4, April, 1980.

26. See Nathan Seppa, "Obesity Research Gets Weightier, *Science News*, 182:13, 12/29/12.

27. Elizabeth Pennisi, "Girth and the Gut," *Science*, vol. 332, 4/1/11.

28. Ibid.

29. Vanessa Ridaura, Jeremiah Faith, et. al., "Gut Microbiota from Twins Discordant for Obesity Modulate Metabolism in Mice," *Science*, vol. 341, 9/16/13.

30. Alan Walker and Julian Parkhill, "Fighting Obesity with Bacteria," *Science*, vol. 341, 9/6/13.

31. See Chin Jou, "The Biology and Genetics of Obesity—A Century of Inquiries," *NEJM*, vol.. 370, 5/15/14, pp. 1874–77.

32. "Of Fat Mice and Men," *Newsweek*, 8/4/52, pp. 52–3.

33. Jou, p. 1876.

34. Joanne Silberner, "Obesity: If the Genes Fit," *Science News*, vol. 129, 1/25/86.

35. Albert Stunkard, Terryl Foch, and Zdenek Hrubec, "A Twin Study of Human Obesity," *JAMA*, 256:1, 7/4/86. More recent estimates place the genetic determinant of obesity at 45–70 percent.

36. "Chubby? Blame Those Genes," *Time*, vol. 135, 6/4/90.

37. Patsy Nishina, "Fifth Obesity Gene Found in Mice" *Science News*, vol. 149, 4/27/96.

38. I. M. Faust, "Surgical Removal of Adipose Tissue Alters Feeding Behavior and the Development of Obesity in Rats," *Science*, vol. 197, 7/22/77. Also, "Obesity Defined" *NEJM*, 274:8, 2/24/66.

39. Jeffrey Freidman, "A War on Obesity, Not the Obese," *Science*, vol. 299, 2/7/03, p. 856–58.

40. Jerry Adler and Mariana Gosnell," "What It Means to Be Fat," *Newsweek*, 12/13/82, p. 84.

41. From Joel Gurin and William Bennett, *The Dieter's Dilemma*, Basic Books, 1983, as quoted in ibid.

42. Quoted in Gina Kolata, "Why It's So Hard to Lose Weight," *Smithsonian*, January, 1986.

43. Denise Grady, "Is Losing Weight a Losing Battle?" *Time*, vol. 131, 3/8/88.

44. Diane Edwards, "Pima Indians: Research by Clifton Bogardus and Others," *Science News*, vol. 132, 11/14/87.

45. Thomas Coates and Carl Thoresen, "Treating Obesity in Children and Adolescents," *AJPH*, 68:2, February, 1978.

46. Quoted in "Of Fat Mice and Men," *Newsweek*, 8/4/52, p. 52.

47. Jack Yanovski, "Recent Advances in Basic Obesity Research," *JAMA*, 282:16, 10/27/99.

48. Coates and Thoresen, "Treating Obesity in Children."

49. Jean Mayer, "The Obese Child," *Today's Education*, January–February, 1974. Also, Anna-Marie Chirico and Albert Stunkard, "Physical Activity and Human Obesity," *NEJM*, 263:19, 11/10/60. Incidentally, Hilda Bruch made similar observations as far back as 1940, noting that most obese children whom she studied were inactive. See Hilda Bruch, "Obesity in Childhood," *Journal of the Disabled Child*, vol. 60, pp. 1082–1109, 1940.

50. See, for example, Jean Mayer, "Decreased Activity and Energy Balance in the Hereditary Obesity-Diabetes Syndrome in Mice," *Science*, vol. 117, 5/8/53.

51. Chirico and Stunkard (1960) note that nearly 100 percent of overweight military recruits who lose weight during the course of basic training regain all of the weight once the training is over.

CHAPTER 3

1. Nagisa Mori, Francisco Armada, and Craig Wilcox, "Walking to School in Japan and Childhood Obesity Prevention: New Lessons from an Old Policy," *AJPH*, 102:11, November 2012, p. 2068–73.

2. The Japanese have a different notion of reasonable walking distance than do Americans. The law requires that elementary schools be placed with four km (2.4 miles) of a child's home and middle schools within six km (3.5 miles). Not only are these distances considered reasonably walkable, but nearly all Japanese children walk to school without parental escort.

3. Jana Hirsch, Ana Diez Roux, et al., "Change in Walking and Body Mass Index Following Residential Relocation: The Multi-Ethnic Study of Atherosclerosis," *AJPH*, 104:3, March 2014, p. e49–56.

4. Y. L Michael, L. A. Perdue, et al., "Physical Activity Resources and Changes in Walking in a Cohort of Older Men," *AJPH*, 100:4, 2010, p. 654–60.

5. About two-thirds of all American domiciles are single-family homes, which is by far the largest proportion in the world.

6. Kenneth Jackson, *The Crabgrass Frontier*, Oxford University Press, 1985, p. 15.

7. *Ibid.*, p. 162.

8. *Ibid.*, p. 163.

9. Wolf von Eckardt, *A Place to Live*, New York, 1974, p. 337; quoted in Jackson, p. 175.

10. Jackson, p. 175.

11. "Flight to the Suburbs," *Time*, 63:12, 3/22/54.

12. The original Levittown Houses, two-bedroom Capes of just under 1,000 square feet, sold for $7,000 in the late 1940s, with no required down payment.

13. Theodore White, "Perspective: 1960," *Saturday Review*, vol. 43, 7/9/60, p 4.

14. Harry Henderson and Sam Shaw, "City to Order," *Collier's*, 2/14/48, p. 17.

15. "Exurbia: It's Not Just a Place, It's This," *Newsweek*, 6/3/57. For a broader treatment of the phenomenon, see Joel Garreau, *Edge City: Life on the New Frontier*, Anchor Books, 1991.

16. Wolfgang Langewiesche, "The Suburbs are Changing," *Reader's Digest*, vol. 95, November 1959, p. 159.

17. Neil Hurley, "The Case for Suburbia," *The Commonweal*, 8/28/59, p. 439.

18. Andres Duany, Elisabeth Plater-Zyberk, and Jeff Speck, *Suburban Nation*, North Point Press, 2000, p. 13.

19. For more, see Robert A. Beauregard, *When America Became Suburban*, University of Minnesota Press, 226. See also, Elizabeth Cohen, *A Consumer's Republic*, Vintage Books, 2003.

20. Deborah Cohen, *Big Fat Crisis*, Nation Books, 2014, p. 172.

21. Quoted in Delores Hayden, *Building Suburbia*, Pantheon, 2003.

22. There is extensive literature of social critique of the ennui, vacuousness, and social conformity of suburban life. For the purposes of this book, I am more interested in the effect of suburban life and landscaping obesity, but interested readers may wish to consult David Riesman, "The Suburban Dislocation," *AAPSS*, vol. 314, November 1957.

23. For an interesting description of Reston, see "A Genial Suburb," *Esquire*, vol. 64, December 1965. For fights over rezoning, see "Battle to Open the Suburbs: New Attack on Zoning Laws," *US News*, 6/22/70. For a more academic take, Peter Siskind, "Suburban Growth and Its Discontents," in Kevin Kruse and Thomas Sugrue, eds., *The New Suburban History*, University of Chicago Press, 2006.

24. Tom Farley and Deborah Cohen, "Fixing a Fat Nation," *Washington Monthly*, 33:12, December 2001.

CHAPTER 4

1. Quoted in Glenna Matthews, *"Just a Housewife": The Rise and Fall of Domesticity in America*, Oxford University Press, 1987, p. 155.

2. Quoted in *ibid.*, p. 157.

3. *Ibid.*, p. 158.

4. Edna Amidon, "Looking Ahead in Vocational Education in Home Economics," *Education for Victory*, 3:17, 3/3/45, p. 6.

5. Phyllis McGinley, "Profession: Housewife," *Ladies Home Journal*, vol. 79, July 1962, p. 10.

6. For example, see Hazel Kory, "Food Purchasing as Affected by Consumer Education," *Journal of Home Economics*, April 1945.

7. Carter Good, "The High School Curriculum in Home Economics," *Journal of Home Economics*, vol. 19, December 1927, as quoted in Rima Apple, "Liberal Arts or Vocational Training?" In Sarah Stage and Virginia Vincenti, eds., *Rethinking Home Economics*, Cornell University Press, 1997.

8. Elizabeth Amery, "Does Home Economics Training Result in Better Home Life?" *Education*, vol. 70, 9/1/49, p. 32.

9. For example, see Sarah Shields Pfeiffer, "He Might like Cooking!" *Parents*, vol. 21, February 1946.

10. Amery, "Does Home Economics Training . . .?", p. 33.

11. Eugenia Smith, "Why I Believe in My Profession," *Practical Home Economics*, vol. 1, May 1956, p. 41.

12. The statistic is from Amitai Etzioni, "The Women's Movement—Tokens vs. Objectives," *Saturday Review*, 5/20/72.

13. Betty Friedan, "Up from the Kitchen Floor," *NYT Magazine*, 3/4/73, p. 8.

14. "Liberation," *New Yorker*, 9/5/70, p. 27.

15. "Sex, Society, and the Female Dilemma," *Saturday Review*, 6/14/75, p. 20.

16. Caroline Moorehead, "A Talk with Simone de Beauvoir," *NYT Magazine*, 6/2/74, p. 22.

17. "Who's Come a Long Way Baby?" *Time*, 96:9, 1970, p. 18.

18. For more, see Susan Brownmiller, "Sisterhood is Powerful," *NYT Magazine*, 3/15/70, p. 230.

19. Mary Segers, "The New Civil Rights: Fem Lib!" *The Catholic World*, August 1970, p. 204.

20. Jane Mansbridge, *Why We Lost the ERA*, University of Chicago Press, 1986.

21. Both quotes are from letters written to feminist Letty Cottin Pogrebin after a television appearance by her. Quoted in Pogrebin, *Family Politics*, McGraw-Hill, 1983, p. 91–92.

22. "Who's Come a Long Way Baby?" p. 20.

23. Quoted in *ibid.* The best description of the league is in Lucianne Goldberg and Jeanne Sakol, *Purr, Baby, Purr*, Pinnacle Books, 1972.

24. Toni Morrison, "What the Black Woman Thinks about Women's Lib," *NYT Magazine*, 8/22/71, p. 15.

25. The statistics are all from Janet Giele, "Decline of the Family: Conservative, Liberal, and Feminist Views," in David Popenoe, Jean Elshtain, and David

Blankenhorn, eds., *Promises to Keep: Decline and Renewal of Marriage in America*, Rowman & Littlefield, 1996.

26. Barbara Dafoe Whitehead, "The Decline of Marriage as the Social Basis for Childrearing," in David Popenoe, Jean Elshtain, and David Blankenhorn, eds., *Promises to Keep: Decline and Renewal of Marriage in America*, Rowman & Littlefield, 1996, p. 8–9.

27. See David Popenoe, *Families without Fathers*, Transaction Publishers, 2009, p. 158–59.

28. Quoted in *ibid.*, p. 162.

29. *Ibid.*, p. 163.

30. Robert Reich, *The Work of Nations*, Alfred Knopf, 1992.

31. Notably, the average workweek fell overall for American workers in the decades after World War II, but this was largely due to greater numbers of part-time workers in the workforce. Full-time workers worked longer weeks.

32. Folke Mossfeldt and Mary Susan Miller, "Don't Just Sit There . . .," *Saturday Evening Post* January/February 1980, p. 56.

33. See Thomas Robinson, "Does Television Cause Childhood Obesity?" *JAMA*, 279:12, 3/25/98, p. 959–60; Robinson, "Reducing Children's Television Viewing to Prevent Obesity: A Randomized Controlled Trial," *JAMA*, 282:16, 10/27/99, p. 1561–67; Gina Kolata, "Obese Children: A Growing Problem," *Science*, vol. 232, 4/4/86, p. 20.

34. Larry Tucker and Marilyn Bagwell, "Television Viewing and Obesity in Adult Females," *AJPH*, 81:7, July 1991, p. 908–11. See also, Tucker and Glenn Friedman, "Television Viewing and Obesity in Adult Males," *AJPH*, 79:4, April 189, p. 516–18.

35. Robert Jeffrey and Simone French, "Epidemic Obesity in the United States: Are Fast Foods and Television Viewing Contributing?" *AJPH*, 88:2, February 1998, p. 277–80.

36. Karen Le Billon, *French Kids Eat Everything*, HarperCollins, 2012, p. 27.

37. Michael Power and Jay Schulkin, *The Evolution of Obesity*, Johns Hopkins University Press, 2009, p. 69.

CHAPTER 5

1. Michael Pollan, *In Defense of Food: An Eater's Manifesto*, Penguin, 2008, p. 7.

2. Ibid., p. 3.

3. For a brilliant history of the evolution in the relationship of farm to city in the nineteenth century, see William Cronon, *Nature's Metropolis: Chicago and the Great West*, Norton, 1991.

4. James Fitch, "When Housekeeping Became a Science," *American Heritage Magazine*, 12:5, 1961.

5. "Dinner Frozen or Dried," *Newsweek*, vol. 26, 11/19/45, pp. 72–74.

6. Elizabeth Beveridge, "Freezing," *Woman's Home Companion*, March 1945, p. 88.

7. Florence Paine, "How Quick Freezing Will Affect Your Future Life," *House Beautiful*, January 1945, p. 63.

8. Ruth Carson, "Food Below Zero," *Collier's*, vol. 115, 1/27/45, p. 48.

9. Jane Holt, "New Shops for Frozen Products," *NYT Magazine*, 7/8/45, p. 26.

10. "Package to Plate—Nonstop!" *Better Homes and Gardens*, June 1945, p. 35.

11. "Dinner, Frozen or Dried," p. 73.

12. See Frederic Nordsiek, "How Processing Affects Nutritive Values of Grain Foods," *AJPH*, vol. 39, June 1949. This a very early study of the effects of bleaching and overmilling on nutrition.

13. James Scheer, "How Food is Sabotaging America," *American Mercury*, vol. 80, May 1955, p. 138.

14. Glenna Matthews, *"Just a Housewife": The Rise and Fall of Domesticity in America*, Oxford University Press, 1987, p. 211.

15. The process of heating organic material with radio waves was discovered in the 1920s and patented by Raytheon in 1945. Commercial microwave ovens were produced in the 1950s, but reasonably priced residential units did not become widespread until 1975.

16. Myrna Johnston, "With Pressure Cooking," *Better Homes and Gardens*, October 1945, p. 37.

17. Pollan points out, to the contrary, that food that can be digested by bacteria can be digested by a human. We should be aware of eating things that microbes find unpalatable!

18. Quoted in Constance Holden, "Food and Nutrition: Is America Due for a National Policy?" *Science*, vol. 184, 5/3/74, p. 550.

19. Elizabeth Abbott, *Sugar: A Bittersweet History*, Penguin, 2008, p. 349.

20. For a more detailed history of the rise of McDonald's, see Eric Schlosser, *Fast Food Nation*, HarperCollins, 2001, particularly pages 18–25.

21. Schlosser, p. 4.

22. Marion Nestle and Michael Jacobson, "Halting the Obesity Epidemic: A Public Health Policy Approach," *PHR*, vol. 115, January/February 2000, pp. 12–24.

23. Brennan Davis and Christopher Carpenter, "Proximity of Fast-Food Restaurants to Schools and Adolescent Obesity," *AJPH*, 99:3, March 2009, pp. 505–10.

24. Quoted in David Kessler, *The End of Overeating*, Rodale Books, 2009, p. 21. I am grateful to Dr. Kessler, a former FDA commissioner, for describing in detail the strategy of these chains in layering fat on salt and on sugar.

25. Ibid.

26. Ibid, p. 77.

27. David Lustig, *Fat Chance*, Plume Books, 2012, p. 57.

28. Philip Elmer-Dewitt, "Fat Times," *Time*, vol. 145, 1/16/95, pp. 58–65.

29. Deborah Cohen, *Big Fat Crisis*, Nation Books, 2014, p. 52.

30. This experiment, and others, are described in ibid., pp. 52–54.

31. See also, Deborah Cohen and Mary Story, "Mitigating the Health Risks of Dining Out: The Need for Standardized Portion Sizes in Restaurants," *AJPH*, 104:4, April 2014, pp. 586–90.

32. Sean Lucan, "Fruit and Vegetable Consumption May Not be Inadequate," *AJPH*, 102:10, October 2012, p. e3.

33. Jennifer Couzin-Frankel, "Tackling America's Eating Habits, One Store at a Time," *Science*, 337:6101, 9/21/12, pp. 1473–75.

34. Ibid., p. 1474. See also Rachel Dannefer, Donya Williams, et al., "Healthy Bodegas: Increasing and Promoting Healthy Foods at Corner Stores in New York City, "*AJPH*, 102:10, October 2012, pp. e27–31.

35. Deborah Cohen, Roland Sturm, et al., "Not Enough Fruit and Vegetables or Too Many Cookies, Candies, Salty Snacks, and Soft Drinks?" *PHR*, 125:1, January–February 2010, p. 88. For a quantitative study on the absence of the food desert effect, see Jessie Handbury, Ilya Rahkovsky, and Molly Schnell, "Is the Focus of Food Deserts Fruitless? Retail Access and Food Purchases across the Socioeconomic Spectrum," 10/9/16, unpublished manuscript.

36. Kessler, *The End of Overeating*, p. 174.

37. Amanda Spake, "A Fat Nation," *US News*, 133:7, 8/19/02, p. 42.

38. Le Billon, *French Kids Eat Everything*, p. 49.

39. The conversation is related in Kessler, *The End of Overeating*, p. 176.

40. Thomas Farley, Erin Baker, et al., "The Ubiquity of Energy-Dense Snack Foods: A National Multicity Study," *AJPH*, 100:2, February 2010, pp. 306–11.

41. Marion Nestle, "Soft Drink 'Pouring Rights': Marketing Empty Calories," *PHR*, vol. 115, July/August 2000, pp. 308–19.

42. Ibid., pp. 311 and 314.

43. Quoted in Spake, "A Fat Nation," p. 43.

44. Cohen, *Big Fat Crisis*, p. 80.

45. Marion Nestle, "Food Marketing and Childhood Obesity—A Matter of Policy," *NEJM*, vol. 354, 6/15/06, pp. 2527–29.

46. Quoted in Steven Spencer, "Are We Overfed but Undernourished?" *Reader's Digest*, vol. 99, 9/1/71, p. 136.

47. Quoted in Nestle, "Pouring Rights," p. 316.

48. Le Billon, *French Kids Eat Everything*, p. 73.

CHAPTER 6

1. "Food and Fat," *Newsweek*, 2/17/47, p. 58.

2. "Obesity Hides Insecurity," *The Science Newsletter*, 52:16, 10/18/47, p. 253.

3. "Obesity the Enemy," *Newsweek*, 10/20/47, p. 54.

4. "The Fat Personality," *Newsweek*, 11/17/52, p. 110.

5. Ibid.

6. "No Laughing Matter," *Newsweek*, 1/31/55, p. 60. Also, Robert Whalen, "We Think Ourselves into Fatness," *NYT Magazine*, 12/3/50; and Russell Maloney, "The Fat of the Land," *Collier's*, 4/10/48.

7. "Overeating Shortens Life," Interview with Fredrick Stare, *US News*, 1/7/55, p. 54

8. Daniel Cappon, *Eating, Loving and Dying: A Psychology of Appetites*, University of Toronto Press, 1973.

9. Laura Beil, "The Snack-Food Trap," *Newsweek*, 160:19, 11/5/12, p. 45.

10. David Kessler, *The End of Overeating*, Rodale, 2009, p. 25.

11. Ibid., p. 26.

12. Ibid., p. 27.

13. Quoted in Carol Pogash, "Of All the Human Frailties, Obesity is the Most Perverse," *Science Digest*, February 1978, p. 59.

14. "Who Gets Fat and Why," *Science Digest*, September 1972.

15. Kessler describes this in *The End of Overeating*, pp. 163–64.

16. Beil, "The Snack-Food Trap."

17. in particular, overeaters were missing D2 receptors, which are responsible for satiation. See Kristin Ozelli, "This is Your Brain on Food," *Scientific American*, 297:3, September 2007.

18. Quoted in Anastasia Toufexis, "Dieting: The Losing Game," *Time*, 1/20/86, pp. 54–60.

19. Neil Rowland and Seymour Antelman, "Stress-Induced Hyperphagia and Obesity in Rats," *Science*, vol. 191, 1/23/76, pp. 310–11.

20. For example, see Robert Carney and Andrew Goldberg, "Weight Gain after Cessation of Cigarette Smoking," *NEJM*, 310:10, 3/8/84, pp.614–16; and Karen Cropsey, Leslie McClure, et al., "The Impact of Quitting Smoking on Weight among Women Prisoners Participating in a Smoking Cessation Intervention," *AJPH*, 100:8, August 2010, pp. 1442–48.

21. For example, see Edward Podolsky, "Angry: You May Need Sugar," *Science Digest*, 7/1/45. See also F. J. Schlink and M. C. Phillips, "Think You Need More Sugar?" *Science Digest*, 5/1/46, condensed from the book, *Meat Three Times a Day*, Richard R Smith Publishers, 1946.

22. Jean Marx, "Cellular Warriors at the Battle of the Bulge," *Science*, 299:5608, 2/7/03, pp. 846–49.

23. See Jean Mayer and Donald Thomas, "Regulation of Food Intake and Obesity," *Science*, vol. 156, 4/21/67, p. 329. See also Donald Coscina and Harvey Stancer, "Selective Blockade of Hypothalmic Lyperphagia and Obesity in Rats by Serotonin-Depleting Midbrain Lesions," *Science*, vol. 195, 1/28/77. In fact, researchers had hypothesized about the role of the hypothalamus from the early

years of the twentieth century, but they had not been able to produce definitive proof.

24. For example, see Michael Schwartz and Daniel Porte Jr., "Diabetes, Obesity, and the Brain," *Science*, vol. 307, 1/21/05, pp. 375–79; see also Schwartz, "Staying Slim with Insulin in Mind," *Science*, 289: 5487, 9/22/00, pp. 2066–67.

25. Robert Lustig writes extensively about this syndrome of leptin suppressions. See his book, *Fat Chance*, Plume Publishers, 2012, particularly pp. 37–60.

26. See work by Kenji Kanagawa and Masayasu Kojima at the National Cardiovascular Center Research Institute in Osaka.

27. Quoted in Marx, "Cellular Warriors," p. 848.

28. Statistics are from "Too Much Sugar," *Consumer Reports*, March 1978, p. 136.

29. Robert Lustig, *Fat Chance*, Plume, 2012, pp. 110–12.

30. Quoted in Nina Teicholz, *The Big Fat Surprise*, Simon and Schuster, 2014, p. 300.

31. The experiment is described in Michael Pollan, *In Defense of Food*, Penguin Press, 2008, pp. 86–87.

32. Described in Ruth Winter, "Are You a Yo-Yo Dieter?" *Science Digest*, vol. 75, 5/1/74, pp. 37–38.

33. "Diabetes: Sugar in the Body," *Science Digest*, vol. 108, 9/13/75, p. 167.

34. For details, see N. L. Jacobson, "The Controversy over the Relationship of Animal Fats to Heart Disease," *BioScience*, vol. 24, 3/1/74, pp. 143–44. Notably, virtually all of the healthier populations lived physically vigorous lives, suggesting that the combination of a sugar-rich diet with a sedentary lifestyle was particularly toxic.

35. "Sugar, Enemy of Good Nutrition," *Consumer Bulletin*, February, 1961. USDA scientists were even skeptical of the replacing tap water with milk!

36. "Teen-Agers are Advised to Eat Starches, Not Sugar," *Science News Letter*, 2/10/62, p. 89.

37. The book was rereleased in 2012. Yudkin's work, initially discredited by the sugar industry and by concerted attacks by Keys, has found renewed acceptance. See Lustig, *Fat Chance*, particularly pp. 110–12.

38. Janet Raloff, "Fructose Risk for High-Fat Diners?" *Science News*, vol. 133, 3/26/88.

39. In 2014, a group of researchers found a correlation between high levels of soda drinking and shortened telomeres in gut cells. Shortened telomeres are correlated with cell aging, suggesting that soft drinks can prematurely age our cells. This study, however, is aberrant; I've seen no others that confirm the finding. See Cindy Leung, Barbara Laraia et al., "Soda and Cell Aging," *AJPH*, 104:12, December 2014, pp. 2425–31.

40. See Harnett Kane, "Revolution in Sugar," *The American Mercury*, vol. 60, March 1945, pp. 310–15. See also Edna Evans, "Sugar Bowl—A Modern

Aladdin's Lamp," *Nature*, vol. 38, May 1945, pp. 233–36. On the American beet industry, George Coons, "The Sugar Beet: Product of Science," *Scientific Monthly*, March 1949.

41. US Representative Paul Findley, R. IL, an arch-foe of protectionism, noted sardonically that subsidies were "very hard to kill, except when the public is fully aroused by exposure to flagrant abuse." See Paul Findley, "Sugar: A Sticky Mess in Congress," *RD*, vol. 88, June 1966, p. 92. See also Boris Swerling, "Sugar and Sympathy," *The Nation*, 2/13/60.

42. "The Sweeteners," TNR, vol. 153, 10/9/65, p. 7.

43. Quoted in "Too Much Sugar?" p. 136.

44. Kathryn Foxhall, "Beginning to Begin: Reports from the Battle on Obesity," *AJPH*, 96:12, December 2006, p. 2106.

45. "Effect of Sugar on Health to be Studied," *Science News*, 5/19/45, p. 319.

46. John Hess, "Harvard's Sugar-Pushing Nutritionist," *Saturday Review*, vol. 5, 8/1/78, pp. 10–14.

47. Quoted in ibid., p 14.

48. For a nice historical summary of diabetes, see Abner Notkins, "The Causes of Diabetes," *Scientific American*, vol. 241, November 1979.

49. Cited in ibid., p. 62.

50. The chain is even more complex. Interested readers are referred to Da Young Oh and Jerrold Olefsky, "Wnt Fans the Flames in Obesity," *Science*, vol. 329, 7/23/10, pp. 397–98; Janet Raloff, "Diabetes: Clarifying the Role of Obesity," *Science News*, vol. 143, 1/2/93; and Joe Alper, "New Insights into Type 2 Diabetes," *Science*, vol. 289, 7/7/00, pp. 37–39.

CHAPTER 7

1. Eileen Burke, "Dieting is No Fun, But . . ." *Today's Health*, 31:1, 3/10/53, p. 42.

2. Ron Chernow, *Alexander Hamilton*, Penguin Books, 2005, p. 333.

3. "Battle of the Bulge," *Time*, 62:6, 8/10/53.

4. Described in Elizabeth Rubin, "New Hope for the Overweight," *Science Digest*, February 1961, p. 39.

5. Quoted in Anastasia Toufexis, "Dieting: The Losing Game," *Time*, vol. 127, 1/20/86, p. 57.

6. "a war with the will," from "The Fat of the Land," *Time*, vol. 77, 1/13/61, p. 49; "an amazing thing," from Amanda Spake, "Stop Dieting!" *US News*, vol. 140, 1/16/06, p. 63.

7. Quoted in Spake, "Stop Dieting," p. 61.

8. See Gina Kolata, "Obese Children: A Growing Problem," *Science*, vol. 232, 4/4/86, p. 21.

9. Quoted in William Mueller, "Of Obesity and Election," *The Christian Century*, 11/26/58, p. 1366.

10. Ibid.

11. "Luncheon Meats, Sausage, Frankfurters, Hamburger," *Consumer Bulletin*, June 1966, p. 23.

12. Harrison Kinney, "President Eisenhower's Special Diet," *McCall's*, December 1957.

13. "What You Should Know about Heart Attacks and High-Fat Diets," *Coronet*, May 1957, pp. 69–70.

14. Ibid.

15. Denise Grady, "Production of Leaner Cattle," *Time*, vol. 131, 4/18/88.

16. Alton Blakeslee, "Can Diet Prevent Heart Attacks?" *Saturday Evening Post*, vol. 237, 1/25/64, p. 66.

17. For example, see Wayne Miller, "Obesity: The Role of Fatty Foods," *Science News*, vol. 138, 10/13/90. See also, James Hill and John Peters, "Environmental Contributions to the Obesity Epidemic," *Science*, vol. 280, 5/29/98.

18. Dean Ornish, *Eat More, Weigh Less*, HarperCollins, 1993.

19. "Facts about Fats," *Current Health*, April 1985, p. 24.

20. Marion Nestle, "The Selling of Olestra," *PHR*, vol. 113, November/December 1998, pp. 508–20.

21. Ibid., p. 517.

22. Robert Bonow and Robert Eckel, "Diet, Obesity, and Cardiovascular Risk," *NEJM*, vol. 348, 5/22/03, pp. 2057–58.

23. Quoted in Nancy Shute, "The Joy of Fat," *US News*, vol. 124, 1/12/98, p. 56.

24. "Fat and Heart Disease," *Time*, vol. 68, 11/12/56.

25. "What You Should Know about Heart Attacks and High-Fat Diets," p. 72.

26. "The Heart: Is Fat at Fault?" *Newsweek*, 5/15/61, p. 92.

27. "Fat, Food, and Heart Disease," *Consumer Reports*, August 1962, p. 411.

28. See "Fat in Diet: The Real Key to Heart Disease?" *Good Housekeeping*, vol. 155, October 1962.

29. Harry Deuel Jr., "The Butter-Margarine Controversy," *Science*, vol. 103, 2/15/46, p. 184.

30. "Eat and Grow Thin," *Newsweek*, 7/18/49, p. 41.

31. See Edgar Gordon, Marshall Goldberg, and Grace Chosy, "A New Concept in the Treatment of Obesity," *JAMA*, 186:1, 10/5/63, pp. 50–60.

32. "Nutrition Program at Cornell: Fatter Cows, Slimmer Women," *Newsweek*, 4/13/53, p. 102. See also, "The High-Fat Diet Fad," *Changing Times*, May 1962, pp. 13–15.

33. "Do Calories Count?" *Consumer Reports*, vol. 27, March 1962, p. 149.

34. Eloise Salholz and Patrice Johnson, "A Diet Doctor's New Prescription," *Newsweek*, 8/22/83, p. 8.

35. M. Smilgis, "Pritikin Will Eat No Fat, Atkins Will Eat No Grain," *People Weekly*, vol. 12, 12/3/79, p. 46.

36. "The High-Fat Diet Fad," p. 14.

37. Ibid., p. 15.

38. "Pritikin Will Eat No Fat," p. 47.

39. S. Boyd Eaton, Marjorie Shostak, and Melvin Konner, *The Paleolithic Prescription*, Harper and Row, 1988. For the AMA's early recommendations, see Clifford Barborka, "Present Status of Obesity Problem," *JAMA*, 147:11, 1951, pp. 1015–19.

40. John Wiley, "Phenomena, Comments, and Notes," *Smithsonian*, October 1988.

41. Quoted in Joel Stein, "The Low-Carb Diet Craze," *Time*, 11/1/99, p. 75.

42. Gary Foster, Holly Wyatt, et al., "A Randomized Trial of Low-Carbohydrate Diet for Obesity," *NEJM*, vol. 348, 5/22/03, pp. 2082–90.

43. "Latest on Being Overweight and What to Do about It," *US News*, 8/28/61.

44. Frederick Stare, "Sense and Nonsense about Nutrition," *Harper's*, vol. 229, October 1964.

45. Gaynor Maddox, "The Ice Cream Diet," *Ladies Home Journal*, vol. 87, September 1970, p. 48. The article is taken from a 1970 book of the same name.

46. "Check Appetite By Eating Less Protein," *Science Digest*, vol. 37, May 1955, p. 22; and, Burr Snider, "Fat City," *Esquire*, vol. 79, March 1973.

47. For anecdotes and reports on (successful) inpatient programs, see the following: W. D. Mogerman, "He Cuts People Down to Size," *Saturday Evening Post*, vol. 228, 12/31/55; Samuel Blondheim, Nathan Kaufmann, and Rachel Poznanski, "The Treatment of Obesity in an Outpatient Dietetic Unit," *JAMA*, 186:12, 12/21/63, pp. 1043–46.The Blondheim/Kaufmann study, at Hadassah Hospital in Jerusalem, combined inpatient and outpatient treatment. The goal of the outpatient component was not to lose weight but to merely maintain the weight loss produced during the inpatient phase.

48. Vincent Dole, "Publicity about 'A Reducing Diet'," *JAMA*, 161:9, 1956, p. 901.

49. H. J. Roberts, "Formula Diets," *JAMA*, 10/21/61.

50. Richard Spark, "Fat Americans," *NYT Magazine*, 2/3/74.

51. Some dieters actually starved to death. See George Mann, "Diet and Obesity," *NEJM*, 4/7/77, p. 812; see also, Judith Willis, "The Fad-Free Diet," *FDA Consumer*, July–August 1985.

52. Quoted in Debby Friss, "The 400 Calorie Solution" *Health*, September 1988, p. 33.

53. "A Macrobiotic Diet That's No Fun and Offers No Proof," *US News*, 2/15/88, p. 75.

54. See George Alexander, "Brown Rice as a Way of Life," *NYT Magazine*, 3/12/72. See also, "The Perils of Eating American Style," *Time*, vol. 100, 12/18/72.

55. "The Most Drastic Way," *Time*, 1/24/64, p. 31. See also, Ernst Drenick, Marion Swendseid, et al., "Prolonged Starvation as Treatment for Severe Obesity," *JAMA*, 187:2, 1/11/64, pp. 100–5; and, "Dramatic Treatment for Obesity: Diseased Patients Test Starvation Diet," *JAMA*, 197:1, 7/4/66, p. 22.

56. See Saul Genuth, Jamie Castro, and Victor Vertes, "Weight Reduction in Obesity by Outpatient Semistarvation," *JAMA*, 230:7, 11/18/74, pp. 987–91.

57. David Stipp, "Is Fasting Good for You?" *Scientific American*, 308:1, January 2013.

58. Interview with W. Henry Sebrell Jr., "What to Eat to Live Longer," *US News*, 4/11/60, p. 92.

59. Frederick Stare, "Bread, Potatoes, Sugar . . .," *McCall's*, vol. 83, January 1956, p. 72.

60. Howard Rusk, "Overweight: Our Primary Health Problem," *NYT*, 11/30/52. Reprinted in *Reader's Digest*, vol. 62, February 1952, p. 124.

61. Harold Aaron, "Weight Control," *Consumer Reports*," vol. 17, February 1952, p. 105. The Rynearson quote may be found in Robert Whalen, "We Think Ourselves into Fatness," *NYT Magazine*, 12/3/50, p. 22.

62. "Weight Control," *JAMA*, 1/19/52, p. 206.

63. "Obesity Anonymous," *Newsweek*, vol. 37, 6/4/51, p. 78; See also Wade Mosby, "Together We Lose," *Today's Health*, April 1955. For a more rigorous analysis of TOPS, see Alfred Rimm, Linda Werner, et al., "Relationship of Obesity and Disease in 73,532 Weight-Conscious Women," *PHR*, 90:1, January–February 1975.

64. "Together We Lose," p. 49.

65. "Obesity Anonymous," p. 78.

66. Lester Breslow, "Public Health Aspects of Weight Control," *AJPH*, vol. 42, September 1952, pp. 1116–20.

67. Helen Lovell, "Weight Reduction Neighborhood Health Program," *JAMA*, 218:7, 11/15/71, p. 1049.

68. Bridget O'Brian, "Who Said Getting Thin is Easy?" *Working Woman*, July 1979, p. 53.

69. Jean Neditch, *The Story of Weight Watchers*, TwentyFirst Corporation Publishers, 1970, p. 27.

70. Thomas Coates and Carl Thoresen, "Treating Obesity in Children and Adolescents," *AJPH*, 68:2, February 1978, pp. 143–51.

CHAPTER 8

1. Quoted in Amanda Spake, "Stop Dieting!" *US News*, 140:2, 1/16/06, p. 61.

2. The example is from "Fat and Unhappy," *Time*, 59:25, 6/23/52.

3. For example, see William Crosby, "Losing Weight through Exercise," *JAMA*, 244:4, 7/25/80, pp. 377–79.

4. Faye Marley, "Winning the Weight Battle," *Science News Letter*, 4/11/64.

5. Jean Mayer, "Exercise Does Keep the Weight Down," *The Atlantic*, vol. 196, 7/1/55, p. 63.

6. Peter Steincrohn, "Exercise after 20? Forget It!" *Science Digest*, 26:5, November 1949, p. 5.

7. Roland Berg, "Exercise Can Help Your Heart," *Look*, vol. 18, 12/14/54.

8. Caroline Bird, "Exercise Can Kill You!" *Cosmopolitan*, vol. 134, June 1953.

9. Quoted in Richard Miller, "Exercise after 40? Yes?" *Science Digest*, November 1950, p. 46.

10. We now know this to be true. See Arthur Snider, "Run for Your Life," *Science Digest*, May 1967, p. 80. For earlier thinking, see "Exercise Makes Hearts Sprout New Arteries," *Science News Letter*, 3/10/56.

11. Matt Clark and Karen Springen, "Running for Your Life," *Newsweek*, 3/12/86, p. 70.

12. Tom Yulsman, "The Scientific Shape-Up," *Science Digest*, August 1984.

13. See Tim Beardsley, "Exercising Choice," *Scientific American*, vol. 260. February 1989.

14. Jean Mayer, "The Best Diet is Exercise," *NYT Magazine*, 4/25/65.

15. George Mann, "The Strange Case of Jack Sprat," *Saturday Evening Post*, vol. 250, March 1978, p. 65.

16. Janice Kaplan, "Fonda On: Fit after Forty," *Vogue*, vol. 175, 2/1/85.

17. Sadly, Fixx died of a heart attack from an undiagnosed congenital condition.

18. Quoted in Harry Waters, "Keeping Fit: America Tries to Shape Up," *Newsweek*, 5/23/78, p. 78.

19. Ibid.

20. From James Fixx, *The Complete Book of Running*, excerpted in "Run Your Way to Happiness," *Reader's Digest*, vol. 113, July 1978, p. 94.

21. "Why 60 Million Americans are on a 'Fitness Kick,'" *US News*, vol. 76, 1/14/74.

22. Recounted in Hal Higdon, "Jogging Is an In Sport," *NYT Magazine*, 4/14/68.

23. Ali Mokdad, Mary Serdula, et al., "The Spread of the Obesity Epidemic in the United States, 1991–1998," *JAMA*, 282:16, 10/27/99, pp. 1519–22.

24. Quoted in Anastasia Toufexis, "The Shape of the Nation," *Time*, vol. 126, 10/7/85, p. 60.

25. "The Progress of Medicine," *Science Digest*, vol. 17, 5/1/45, p. 48.

26. Walter Modell, "Status and Prospect of Drugs for Overeating," *JAMA*, 173:10, 7/9/60, pp. 1131–36.

27. "Cigarettes for Reducing," *Consumer Reports*, vol. 23, August 1958.

28. Roger Jelliffe, Dennis Hill, et al., "Death from Weight-Control Pills," *JAMA*, 208:10, 6/9/69, p. 1843.

29. Rita Rubin, "When Willpower Won't," *US News*, vol. 118, 5/15/95.

30. Michael Davidson, Jonathan Hauptman, et al., "Weight Control and Risk Factor Reduction in Obese Subjects Treated for 2 Years with Orlistat," *JAMA*, 281:3, 1/20/99, pp. 235–42. See also, Trisha Gura, "Obesity Drug Pipeline Not So Fat," *Science*, vol. 299, 2/7/03, pp. 849–852.

31. Erica Westly, "Fat Attack," *Scientific American*, 303:3, September 2010.

32. Maria Farina, Roberto Baratta, et al., "Intragastric Balloon in Association with Lifestyle and/or Pharmacotherapy in the Long-Term Management of Obesity," *Obesity Surgery*, vol. 22, 2012, pp. 565–71.

33. John Elliot, "More Help for the Morbidly Obese: Gastric Stapling," *JAMA*, 240:18, 10/27/78, p. 1941.

34. Hans-Rudolf Berthoud, "Why Does Gastric Bypass Surgery Work?" *Science*, 341:6144, 7/26/13, pp. 351–52.

35. Joan Briscoe, "I Chose Surgery to Lose Weight," *Good Housekeeping*, vol. 176, May 1973, p. 56. See also, L. A. Lewis, "Short-Circuiting of Small Intestine," *JAMA*, vol. 182, 1962, pp. 77–79; and Ronald Malt and Frederick Guggenheim, "Surgery for Obesity," *NEJM*, 295:1, 7/1/76, pp. 43–44.

36. Eric DeMaria, "Bariatric Surgery for Morbid Obesity," *NEJM*, vol. 356, 5/24/07, pp 2176–83.

37. Colleen Rand, John Kuldau, and Lynn Robbins, "Surgery for Obesity and Marriage Quality," *JAMA*, 247:10, 3/12/82, pp. 1419–22.

38. American Society for Metabolic and Bariatric Surgery, "New Evidence Prompts Update to Metabolic and Bariatric Surgery Guidelines," downloaded from https://asmbs.org/articles/new-evidence-prompts-update-to-metabolic-and-bariatric-surgery-guidelines, 2/1/17.

39. Elizabeth Pennisi, "Girth and the Gut (Bacteria)," *Science*, 332:6025, 4/1/11, pp. 32–33.

40. Laura Cox and Martin Blaser, "Antibiotics in Early Life and Obesity," *National Review of Endocrinology*, 11:3, March 2015, pp. 182–90.

41. Tine Jess, "Microbiota, Antibiotics, and Obesity," *NEJM*, vol. 371, 12/25/14, pp. 2526–28.

42. Vanessa Ridaura, Jeremy Faith, et al., "Cultured Gut Microbiota from Twins Discordant for Obesity Modulate Adiposity and Metabolic Phenotypes in Mice," *Science*, vol. 341, 9/6/13.

43. Alan Walker and Julian Parkhill, "Fighting Obesity with Bacteria," *Science*, 341:6150, 9/6/13, pp. 1069–70.

44. Mara Hvistendahl, "My Microbiome and Me," *Science*, 336:6086, 6/8/12, pp. 1248–50.

45. The earliest mention I could find was an untitled piece by Ruth Okay and Dorothy Stewart in *Journal of Biological Chemistry*, vol. 99, February 1933, p. 717. Rudolf Virchow noted deposits of fatty arterial plaques in nineteenth-century autopsies, at the time called "atheromata."

46. Steven Spencer, "Are You Eating Your Way to a Heart Attack," *Saturday Evening Post*, vol. 229, 12/1/56.

47. Caroline Thomas and Stanley Garn, "Degree of Obesity and Serum Cholesterol Level," *Science*, vol. 131, 9/19/59, p. 42.

48. "Calories More Than Fat Control Artery Disease," *Science News Letter*, 2/27/54, p. 136.

49. "Butter to Spare Arteries," *Science News Letter*, 4/28/56, p. 261.

50. Solid plant fats could either be artificially hydrogenated, as in the case of Crisco and most margarines, or they could be naturally solid, such as those derived from palm and coconut.

51. N. L. Jacobson, "The Controversy over the Relationship of Animal Fats to Heart Disease," *BioScience*, 24:3, March 1974, pp. 141–48.

52. Madeleine Nash, "Is a Low Fat Diet Risky?" *Time*, vol. 144, 9/5/94.

53. The product flopped. See Vic Sussman, "A Fresh Attack on Red Meat," *US News*, vol. 109, 12/31/90.

54. Angela Haupt, "Try a New Twist on the Atkins Diet," *US News*, 147:11, December 2010, p. 17.

CHAPTER 9

1. For a discussion of a number of similar experiments in the 1960s and 1970s on self-control, see Walter Mischel, Yuichi Shoda, and Monica Rodriguez, "Delay of Gratification in Children," *Science*, 244:4907, 5/26/89, pp. 933–38.

2. See John Tierney, "Do You Suffer from Decision Fatigue?" *NYT Magazine*, 8/17/11.

3. Roy Baumeister had done extensive work in ego depletion and coined the term. See note 4.

4. See Roy Baumeister, Ellen Bratslavsky, Mark Muraven, and Dianne Tice, "Ego Depletion: Is the Active Self a Limited Resource?" *Journal of Personality and Social Psychology*, 74:5, May 1998, pp. 1252–65. See also, Daniel Kahneman, "A Perspective on Judgment and Choice," *American Psychologist*, 58:9, September 2003, pp. 697–720.

5. Matthew Gailliot, Roy Baumeister, et al., "Self-Control Relies on Glucose as a Limited Energy Source: Willpower is More Than a Metaphor," *Journal of Personality and Social Psychology*, 92:2, February 2007, pp. 325–36.

6. Tierney, "Do You Suffer from Decision Fatigue?", p. 6. Tierney notes that the decision with regards to planning a wedding constitutes the decision-fatigue equivalent of "Hell Week."

7. See Deborah Cohen and Susan Babey, "Candy at the Cash Register: A Risk Factor for Obesity and Chronic Disease," *NEJM*, vol. 367, 10/11/12, pp. 1381–83.

8. Europeans are puzzled by the corporate practice in the United States of catering business meetings. One Dutch executive reflected, "We go to a meeting in America and somebody will inevitably bring in a huge plate of bagels and cream cheese and muffins and all of these things. For Europeans, it comes off as bizarre." From David Kessler, *The End of Overeating*, Rodale Books, 2009.

9. Stanley Schachter, "Obesity and Eating: Internal and External Cues Differentially Affect the Eating Behavior of Obese and Normal Subjects," *Science*, 161:3843, 8/23/68, pp. 751–56.

10. Ibid., p. 751.

11. Richard Spark, "Fat Americans," *NYT Magazine*, 1/6/74, p. 42.

12. See Deborah Cohen and Mary Story, "Mitigating the Health Risks of Dining Out: The Need for Standardized Portion Sizes in Restaurants," *AJPH*, 104:4, April 2014, pp. 586–90.

13. Kiera Butler, "Let Them Eat Junk," *Mother Jones*, 40:2, March/April 2015.

14. Susan Yanovski, "Obesity Treatment in Primary Care—Are We There Yet?" *NEJM*, vol. 365, 11/24/11, pp. 2030–31.

15. Alice Lake, "Take Pounds off—and Keep Them off—with Behavior Therapy," *McCall's,* 1972.

16. Hall Currey, Robert Malcolm, et al., "Behavioral Treatment of Obesity," *JAMA*, 237:26, 6/27/77. For more recent work, see Thomas Wadden, Meghan Butryn, et al., "Behavioral Treatment of Obesity in Patients Encountered in Primary Settings," *JAMA*, 312:17, 11/5/14, pp. 1779–91.

17. See David Freedman, "How to Fix the Obesity Crisis," *Scientific American*, 304:2, February 2011.

18. "Drugs and Obesity," *JAMA*, 204:4, 4/22/68, p. 118.

19. Maia Szalavitz, "Can You Get Over an Addiction?" *NYT*, 6/26/16.

20. Gina Kolata, *Rethinking Thin*, Farrar, Straus, and Giroux, 2007, pp. 10–16.

21. Quoted in Amanda Spake, "The Science of Slimming," *US News*, vol. 134, 6/16/03, p. 36.

22. The Mann research is summarized in "What Fights Fat Best?" *Science Digest*, November 1974, pp. 48–9.

23. See David Freedman, "How to Fix the Obesity Crisis," *Scientific American*, 304:2, February 2011.

24. See Kessler, p. 177.

25. See Olga Khazan, "Why Rich Women Don't Get Fat," *Atlantic Monthly*, 313:3, April 2014.

26. Rod Dishman, James Sallis, and Diane Orenstein, "The Determinants of Physical Activity and Exercise," *PHR*, 100:2, March–April 1985, pp. 158–71.

27. Ibid., p. 166.

28. Hanna Rosin, "The Fat Tax," *The New Republic*, 218:20, 5/18/98.

29. Geoffrey Cowley, "Generation XXL," *Newsweek*, 136:1, 7/3/00.

30. Rafael Claro, Renata Levy, et al., "Sugar-Sweetened Beverage Taxes in Brazil," *AJPH*, 102:1, January 2012, pp. 178–83.

31. Jason Block, Amitabh Chandra, et al., "Point-of-Purchase Price and Education Intervention to Reduce Consumption of Sugary Soft Drinks," *AJPH*, 100:8, August 2010, pp. 1427–33.

32. M. J. Friedrich, "Tax on Sugary Beverages in India Could Reduce Obesity and Diabetes," *JAMA*, 311:7, 2014, p. 666.

33. Quoted in Wendy Mariner and George Annas, "Limiting 'Sugary Drinks' to Reduce Obesity—Who Decides?" *NEJM*, vol. 368, 5/9/13, pp. 1763–65.

34. Lawrence Gostin, Belinda Reeve, and Marice Ashe, "The Historic Role of Boards of Health in Local Innovation: New York City's Soda Portion Case," *JAMA*, 312:15, October 2014, pp. 1511–12.

35. James Surowiecki, "Downsizing Supersize," *New Yorker*, 88:24, 8/13/12, p. 36.

36. Scot Burton, Elizabeth Creyer, et al., "Attacking the Obesity Epidemic: The Potential Health Benefits of Providing Nutrition Information in Restaurants," *AJPH*, 96:9, September 2006, pp. 1669–75.

CHAPTER 10

1. Irina Grafova, Vicki Freedman, et al., "Neighborhoods and Obesity in Later Life," *AJPH*, 98:11, November 2008, p. 392.

2. The literature is extensive. For example, see Anne Wolf, Steven Gortmaker, et al., "Activity, Inactivity, and Obesity: Racial, Ethnic, and Age Differences among Schoolgirls," *AJPH*, 83:11, November 1993, pp. 1625–27.

3. Philip Elmer-Dewitt, "Fat Times," *Time*, vol. 145, 1/16/95. See also Diane Edwards, "Metabolism Studies Predict Obesity," *Science News*, vol. 132, 11/14/87.

4. Helen Margellos-Anast, Ami Shah, and Steve Whitman, "Prevalence of Obesity among Children in Six Chicago Communities," *PHR*, 123:2, March–April 2008, pp. 117–25.

5. Lisa Bates, Dolores Acevedo-Garcia, et al., "Immigration and Generational Trends in Body Mass Index and Obesity in the United States," *AJPH*, 98:1, January 2008, pp. 70–78.

6. This effect has been known for fifty years. See Helen Morioka and Myrtle Brown, "Incidence of Obesity and Overweight among Honolulu Police and Firemen," *PHR*, 85:5, May 1970, pp. 433–39.

7. Jennifer Tang, "The First in the Family to be Supersized," *Newsweek*, 148:6, 8/7/06, p. 18.

8. Stanley Garn, "Obesity in Black and White Mothers and Daughters," *AJPH*, 84:11, November 1994, pp. 1727–28.

9. Gary Taubes, "As Obesity Rates Rise, Experts Struggle to Explain Why," *Science*, 280:5368, 5/29/98, pp. 1367–68.

10. Sherman James, Angela Fowler-Brown, et al., "Life-Course Socioeconomic Position and Obesity in African American Women," *AJPH*, 96:3, March 2006, pp. 554–60; See also Daniel Hruschka, Alexandra Brewis, et al., "Shared Norms and Their Explanation for the Social Clustering of Obesity," *AJPH*, 101:supp. 1, December 2011, pp. S295–300.

11. Mir Ali, John Rizzo, and Frank Heiland, "Big and Beautiful? Evidence of Racial Difference in the Perceived Attractiveness of Obese Females," *Journal of Adolescence*, vol. 36, 2013, p. 547.

12. Margaret Hicken, Hedwig Lee, et al., "Racial/Ethnic Disparities in Hypertension Prevalence," *AJPH*, 104:1, January 2014, p. 118.

13. James Kirby, Lan Liang, et al., "Race, Place, and Obesity: The Complex Relationships among Community Racial/Ethnic Composition, Individual Race/Ethnicity, and Obesity in the United States," *AJPH*, 102:8, August 2012, pp. 1572–78.

14. See James Burns, Sarah Goff, et al., "The Relationship between Local Food Sources and Open Space to Body Mass Index in Urban Children," *PHR*, 126:6, November–December 2011, pp. 890–900.

15. Parvez Hossain, Bisher Kawar, and Meguid El Nahas, "Obesity and Diabetes in the Developing World—A Growing Challenge," *NEJM*, vol. 356, 1/18/07, pp. 213–15.

16. Barry Popkin "The World is Fat," *Scientific American*, 297:3, September, 2007.

17. Ivan Pawson and Craig Janes, "Massive Obesity in a Migrant Samoan Population," *AJPH*, 71:5, May 1981, pp. 508–13.

18. Bradford Lowell and Gerald Shulman, "Mitochondrial Dysfunction and Type 2 Diabetes," *Science*, 307:5708 1/21/05, pp. 384–87.

19. Sasiragha Reddy, Ken Resnicow, et al., "Rapid Increases in Overweight and Obesity among South African Adolescents," *AJPH*, 102:2, February 2012, pp. 262–68.

20. Carlow Monteiro, Wolney Conde, and Barry Popkin, "Income-Specific Trends in Obesity in Brazil: 1975–2003," *AJPH*, 97:10, October 2007, pp. 1808–12.

21. Wayne Millar and Thomas Stephens, "The Prevalence of Overweight and Obesity in Britain, Canada, and the United States," *AJPH*, 77:1, January 1987, pp. 38–41.

22. Gary Taubes, "Weight Increases Worldwide?" *Science*, 280:5368, 5/29/98, pp. 1368.

23. Mary Moore, Albert Stunkard, et al., "Obesity, Social Class, and Mental Illness," *JAMA*, 181:11, 9/15/62, 503–8. See also Stacey Rosen and Shahla Shapouri, "Obesity in the Midst of Unyielding Food Insecurity in Developing Countries," *Amber Waves*, 6:4, September 2008.

24. Phillip Goldblatt, Mary Moore, and Albert Stunkard, "Social Factors in Obesity," *JAMA*, 192:12, 6/21/65, pp. 1039–44.

25. Albert Stunkard, Eugene d'Aquili, et al., "Influence of Social Class on Obesity and Thinness in Children," *JAMA*, 221:6, 8/7/72, pp. 579–84; See also Soveig Cunningham, Michael Kramer, and Venkat Narayan, "Incidence of Childhood Obesity in the United States," *NEJM*, vol. 370, 1/30/14, pp. 403–11.

26. "Fat People's Fight against Job Bias," *US News*, 12/5/77.

27. Helen Canning and Jean Mayer, "Obesity—Its Possible Effect on College Acceptance," *NEJM*, 275:21, 11/24/66, p. 1172.

28. "Discrimination: Weighty Problem," *Newsweek*, 3/31/75.

29. See Gina Kolata, "Obesity Declared a Disease," *Science*, 227:4690, 3/1/85, pp. 1019–20.

30. Michelle Stacey, "Let Them Eat Cake," *NYT Magazine*, 12/17/95, p. 51.

31. Laura Shapiro, "Fat Times at Ridgemont High," *Newsweek*, vol. 122, 11/8/93, p. 75.

32. Lorraine Reitzel, Seann Regan, et al., "Density and Proximity of Fast Food Restaurants and Body Mass Index among African Americans," *AJPH*, 104:1, January 2014, pp. 110–16.

33. Susan Babey, Theresa Hastert, et al., "Income Disparities in Obesity Trends among California Adolescents," *AJPH*, 100:11, November 2010, pp. 2149–55.

34. Chandra Tiwary and Alfonso Holguin, "Prevalence of Obesity among Children of Military Dependents at Two Major Medical Centers," *AJPH*, 82:3, March 1992, pp. 354–57.

35. Claire Maturo and Solveig Cunningham, "Influence of Friends on Children's Physical Activity: A Review," *AJPH*, 103:7, July 2013, pp. e23–38.

36. David Schaefer and Sandra Simpkins, "Using Social Network Analysis to Clarify the Role of Obesity in Selection of Adolescent Friends," *AJPH*, 104:7, July 1014, pp. 1223–29.

37. Nicholas Christakis and James Fowler, "The Spread of Obesity in a Large Social Network over 32 Years," *NEJM*, vol. 357, 7/26/07, pp. 370–79.

38. Ibid.

39. Luise Franzini, Marc Elliott, et al., "Influences of Physical and Social Neighborhood Environments on Children's Physical Activity and Obesity," *AJPH*, 99:2, February 2009, pp. 271–78.

40. Eileen Burke, "Dieting is No Fun, But . . ." *Today's Health*, 1/1/53, p. 70.

41. Joseph Marks, "Is Your Family Making You Fat?" *Science Digest*, July 1975, p. 67.

42. John Neill, John Marshall, and Charles Yale, "Marital Changes after Intestinal Bypass Surgery," *JAMA*, 240:5, 8/4/78, p. 448.

43. Ibid., p. 449.

CHAPTER 11

1. Rebecca Voelker, "Escalating Obesity Rates Pose Health, Budget Threats," *JAMA*, 308:15, 10/17/12, p. 1514. On the recent plateauing of obesity rates, see Susan Yanovski and Jack Yanovski, "Obesity Prevalence in the United States—Up, Down, or Sideways?" *NEJM*, vol. 364, 3/17/11, pp. 987–89.

2. Jennifer Cross, "The Politics of Food," *The Nation*, 8/17/74, p. 114.

3. For more on the evolution of the human body, see Daniel Lieberman, *The Story of the Human Body*, Pantheon, 2013.

4. Kenneth Krause, "Saving Us from Sweets," *Skeptical Inquirer*, 36:5, September–October, 2012, p. 24.

5. See Deborah Cohen and Mary Story, "Mitigating the Health Risks of Dining Out: The Need for Standardized Portion Sizes in Restaurants," *AJPH*, 104:4, April 2014, pp. 586–90.

6. Tom Farley and Deborah Cohen, "Fixing a Fat Nation," *Washington Monthly*, 33:12, December 2001, p. 23.

7. One study demonstrated that in a typical PE class children spent less than 10 percent of the period actually moving vigorously. See Rosemary Flores "Dance for Health: Improving Fitness in African American and Hispanic Adolescents," *PHR*, 110:2, March–April 1995, pp. 189–93. Also, B. G. Simons-Morton, W. C. Taylor, et al., "The Physical Activity of Fifth-Grade Students during Physical Education Classes," *AJPH*, vol. 83, 1993, pp. 262–64.

8. Susan Okie, "New York to Trans Fats: You're Out!" *NEJM*, vol. 356, 5/17/07, pp. 2017–22.

9. See John Amis, Paul Wright, et al., "Implementing Childhood Obesity Policy in a New Educational Environment: The Cases of Mississippi and Tennessee," *AJPH*, 102:7, July 2012., pp. 1406–13.

10. Margaret Deirdre O'Hartigan, "The Joy of Fat," *Harper's*, vol. 288, May 1994, p. 40.

11. From Leonard Engel, "Do We Have to Give Up Smoking?" *Harper's*, vol. 209, 12/1/54.

12. E. Cuyler Hammond, "The Effects of Smoking," *Scientific American*, 207:1, July 1962.

13. "Cigarettes," *Consumer Reports*, March 1957, p. 108. The article was drawn largely for the American Cancer Society report authored by E. Cuyler Hammond and Daniel Horn.

14. Ibid., p. 109.

15. Quoted in, "Can You Smoke and Keep Your Health?" *Consumer Bulletin*, July 1958, p. 13.

16. "The Danger of Smoking: More than Cancer," *Time*, 80:1, 7/6/62.

17. The original report may be downloaded from https://profiles.nlm.nih.gov/ps/access/nnbbmq.pdf.

18. John Blatnik, "Making Cigarette Ads Tell the Truth," *Harper's*, August 1958, p. 45.

19. The quote is from Charles Kensler, a cancer researcher who did early work on charcoal filters. See "Will Science Find a Safer Cigarette?" *Popular Science*, July 1964, p. 162.

20. "Smoking Scare? What's Happened to It," *UN News*, 1/11/65.

21. Bill Davidson, "New Hope for Cigarette Smokers: Crash Effort for a Safer Cigarette," *Saturday Evening Post*, vol. 273, 4/18/64.

22. Alastair Burnet, "Smoking May Produce Cancer; It Also Produces Revenue," *The New Republic*, 5/7/62.

23. "The Smoking Report and Advertising Ethics," *America*, 1/25/64, p. 132.

24. Thomas Whiteside, "Smoking Still," *New Yorker*, 11/18/74, p. 121.

25. James Colbert and Jonathan Adler, "Sugar-Sweetened Beverages," *NEJM*, vol. 368, 1/17/13.

26. Nick Sibilla, "Baking Bad: Selling Homemade Cakes and Cookies Could Mean Criminal Penalties in Wisconsin," *Forbes*, 1/26/16.

Selected Bibliography

Abbot, Elizabeth. *Sugar: A Bittersweet History*. New York: Overlook Press, 2011.

Ackerman, Frank, Neva Goodwin, Laurie Dougherty, and Kevin Gallagher, eds. *The Changing Nature of Work*. Washington, DC: Island Press, 1998.

Ariely, Dan. *Predictably Irrational*. New York: HarperCollins, 2008.

Bailey, Eric. *Food Choice and Obesity in Black America*. New York: Praeger, 2006.

Banks, Ralph Richard. *Is Marriage for White People?* New York: Plume, 2012.

Beauregard, Robert. *When America Became Suburban*. Minneapolis: University of Minnesota Press, 2006.

Bell, Kirsten, Amy Salmon, and Darlen McNaughton. *Alcohol, Tobacco, and Obesity*. London: Routledge, 2012.

Bennett, Constance and Stephen Sinatra. *Sugar Shock*. Berkley, CA: Berkley Publishing Group, 2006.

Bernard, Richard and Bradley Rice. *Sunbelt Cities*. Austin: University of Texas Press, 1983.

Borstelmann, Thomas. *The 1970s*. Princeton, NJ: Princeton University Press, 2013.

Brandt, Allan. *The Cigarette Century*. New York: Basic Books, 2009.

Braunstein, Peter and Michael Doyle, eds. *Imagine Nation*. London: Routledge, 2001.

Cohen, Deborah. *A Big Fat Crisis*. New York: Nation Books, 2014.

Crawford, Matthew. *Shop Class as Soulcraft*. New York: Penguin, 2010.

Duany, Andres, Elizabeth Plater-Zyberk, and Jeff Speck. *Suburban Nation*. New York: North Point Press, 2010.

Foxcroft, Louise. *Calories and Corsets*. London: Profile, 2013.

Freedman, Estelle. *No Turning Back.* New York: Ballantine, 2003.

Frymer, Paul. *Black and Blue.* Princeton, NJ: Princeton University Press, 2007.

Garcia, Guy. *The Decline of Men.* New York: Harper, 2009.

Garreu, Joel. *Edge City.* New York: Anchor, 1992.

Gillespie, David. *Sweet Poison.* New York: Penguin, 2009.

Griffiths, Sian and Jennifer Wallace, eds. *Consuming Passion.* Manchester: Mandolin, 1998.

Guiliano, Mireille. *French Women Don't Get Fat.* New York: Vintage, 2007.

Harrald, Chris and Fletcher Watkins. *The Cigarette Book.* New York: Skyhorse, 2010.

Hayden, Dolores. *Building Suburbia.* New York: Vintage, 2004.

Heery, Edmund and John Salmon, eds. *The Insecure Workforce.* London: Routledge, 2000.

Hise, Greg. *Magnetic Los Angeles.* Baltimore: Johns Hopkins University Press, 1999.

Jackson, Ken. *Crabgrass Frontier.* New York: Oxford University Press, 1987.

Jacobs, Jane. *The Death and Life of Great American Cities.* New York: Vintage, 1992.

Jakle, John and Keith Sculle. *Fast Food.* Baltimore: Johns Hopkins University Press, 1999.

Kessler, David. *The End of Overeating.* Emmaus, PA: Rodale, 2009.

Kluger, Richard. *Ashes to Ashes.* New York: Vintage, 1996.

Kolata, Gina. *Rethinking Thin.* New York: Farrar, Straus and Giroux, 2007.

Kruse, Kevin and Thomas Sugrue, eds. *The New Suburban History.* Chicago: University of Chicago Press, 2006.

Kunstler, James Howard. *The Geography of NoWhere.* New York: Free Press, 1994.

Le Billon, Karen. *French Kids Eat Everything.* Boston: Little, Brown, 2012.

Levine, Susan. *School Lunch Politics.* Princeton, NJ: Princeton University Press, 2008.

Levitt, Steven and Steven Dubbner. *Freakonomics.* New York: HarperCollins, 2009.

Lieberman, Daniel. *The Story of the Human Body.* New York: Pantheon, 2013.

Lindop, Edmund. *America in the 1950s.* New York: Twenty-First Century Books, 2009.

Love, Barbara, ed. *Feminists Who Changed America.* Urbana, IL: University of Illinois Press, 2006.

Lustig, Robert. *Fat Chance.* New York: Plume, 2013.

Marsden, George. *The Twilight of the American Enlightenment.* New York: Basic Books, 2014.

Matthews, Glenna. *Just a Housewife.* New York: Oxford University Press, 1987.

Matusow, Allen. *The Unraveling of America.* Athens, GA: University of Georgia Press, 2009.

Monteith, Sharon. *American Culture in the 1960s*. Edinburgh: Edinburgh University Press, 2008.

Moss, Michael. *Salt, Sugar, Fat*. New York: Random House, 2014.

Murray, Charles. *Coming Apart*. New York: Crown, 2012.

Nidetch, Jean and Joan Heilman. *The Story of Weight Watchers*. New York: Signet, 1972.

Packer, George. *The Unwinding*. New York: Farrar, Straus and Giroux, 2013.

Pearlstein, Mitch. *From Family Collapse to America's Decline*. Lanham: Rowman & Littlefield, 2011.

Pollan, Michael. *In Defense of Food*. New York: Penguin, 2008.

Popenoe, David, Jean Bethke Elshtain, and David Blankenhorn. *Promises to Keep*. Lanham: Rowman & Littlefield, 1996.

Popenoe, David. *Disturbing the Nest*. Piscataway, NJ: Transaction Publishers, 1988.

Popenoe, David. *Families without Fathers*. Piscataway, NJ: Transaction Publishers, 2009.

Power, Michael and Jay Schulkin. *The Evolution of Obesity*. Baltimore: Johns Hopkins University Press, 2009.

Putnam, Robert. *Bowling Alone*. New York: Simon & Schuster, 2000.

Rifkin, Jeremy. *The End of Work*. New York: Tarcher, 1996.

Rochefort, Harriet. *French Toast*. New York: St. Martin's Press, 1997.

Rosin, Hanna. *The End of Men: And the Rise of Women*. New York: Riverhead, 2012.

Schlosser, Eric. *Fast Food Nation*, Boston: Houghton Mifflin, 2001.

Schultz, Nick. *Home Economics*. Washington, DC: AEI Press, 2013.

Schwartz, Hillel. *Never Satisfied*. New York: Diane, 2007.

Smith, Andrew. *Food and Drink in American History*. Santa Barbara: ABC-CLIO, 2013.

Stage, Sarah and Virginia Vincenti, eds. *Rethinking Home Economics*. Ithaca, NY: Cornell University Press, 1997.

Stewart, James, ed. *African Americans and Post-Industrial Labor Markets*. London: Routledge, 1997.

Sutherland, Stuart. *Irrationality*. London: Pinter & Martin, 2013.

Teicholz, Nina. *The Big Fat Surprise*. New York: Simon & Schuster, 2014.

Tiger, Lionel. *The Decline of Males*. New York: St. Martin's Press, 2000.

Wilkinson, Alec. *Big Sugar*. New York: Knopf, 1989.

Yudkin, John. *Pure, White, and Deadly*. New York: Penguin, 1972.

Index

About the Author

Jonathan Engel writes about the historical evolution of US health and social welfare policy. His books are *Doctors and Reformers: Discussion and Debate over Health Policy, 1925–1950* (2002); *Poor People's Medicine: Medicaid and American Charity Care since 1965* (2006); *The Epidemic: A Global History of AIDS* (2006); *American Therapy: The Rise of Psychotherapy in the United States* (2008); and *Unaffordable: American Healthcare from Johnson to Trump* (2018). Engel is a professor at the Marxe School of Public and International Affairs, CUNY. In addition, he has taught at the Mailman School of Public Health at Columbia University and the School of Public Health at the University of Massachusetts.